RENAL DIET COOKBOOK 2024

Simple delicious recipes, including nutritional information, health advantage, 14 days meal plan, and more.

JOHN M. VALENZUELA

Copyright © 2024 John M. Valenzuela

All right reserved.

No part of this publication may be reproduced, distributed, or transmitted in any form or by any means, including photocopying, recording, or other electronic or mechanical methods, without the prior written permission of the publisher, except in the case of quotations embodied in critical reviews and certain other noncommercial uses permitted by copyright law.

Legal & disclaimer

The contents and information contained in this book has been compiled from reliable sources, which are accurate based on the knowledge, belief, expertise and information of the Author. The author cannot be held liable for any omissions and/or errors.

CONTENT

INTRODUCTION 1
Understanding the Renal Diet 1
Benefits of a Renal Diet 3
Essential Nutrients and Restrictions in a Renal Diet 5
BREAKFAST 9
Low-Phosphorus Pancakes 10
Herb-Infused Egg White Omelet 12
Cinnamon Quinoa Porridge 14
2 16
LIGHT AND FRESH SALAD 16
Cucumber Dill Salad 17
Berry Spinach Salad with Lemon Vinaigrette 19
Zesty Quinoa and Veggie Salad 21
SAVORY SOUPS AND STEWS 23
Hearty Vegetable Soup 24
Chicken and Rice Soup 26
Lentil and Sweet Potato Stew 28
DELICIOUS MAIN COURSES 30
Herb-Crusted Baked Cod 30
Grilled Lemon Chicken 33
Vegetarian Stuffed Peppers 35
Garlic and Herb Pork Tenderloin 38
Zucchini Noodles with Pesto 40
SATISFYING SIDES 42
Roasted Brussels Sprouts with Lemon 43
Garlic Mashed Cauliflower 45
Spicy Roasted Carrots 47
Quinoa Pilaf with Herbs 49
SNACK TIME 51
Baked Kale Chips 51

Spicy Chickpea Snack 54
Apple Slices with Almond Butter 56
SMOOTHIES AND BEVERAGES 59
Green Detox Smoothie 60
Berry Banana Smoothie 62
Herbal Iced Tea 64
HEAlthy DESSERTS 66
Baked Apple with Cinnamon 67
Vanilla Chia Seed Pudding 69
Rice Pudding with Nutmeg 71
Berry Sorbet 73
INTERNATIONAL FLAVORS 75
Mediterranean Chicken Skewers 76
Asian-Inspired Stir-Fry 78
Mexican-Style Tofu Tacos 81
Indian Spiced Lentils 84
10 86
COMFORT FOOD MAKEOVERS 86
Cauliflower Mac and Cheese 86
Turkey Meatloaf 89
Low-Sodium Beef Stroganoff 91
Chicken Pot Pie with a Twist 94
SPECIAL OCCASION MEALS 97
Rosemary Lamb Chops 97
Stuffed Chicken Breast with Spinach and Cheese 100
Seared Scallops with Lemon Butter 103
MEAL PLAN 105
CONCLUSION 108

INTRODUCTION

Understanding the Renal Diet

The renal diet, often recommended for individuals with chronic kidney disease (CKD) or those undergoing dialysis, is a specialized eating plan designed to support kidney function and prevent further damage. This diet focuses on managing the intake of specific nutrients and minerals that can burden the kidneys, thereby helping to maintain overall health and well-being.

The Role of Kidneys in the Body

Before delving into the specifics of the renal diet, it's essential to understand the critical functions of the kidneys:

- **Filtering Waste**: Kidneys filter waste products and excess fluids from the blood, excreting them through urine.
- **Balancing Electrolytes**: They help maintain the balance of electrolytes such as sodium, potassium, and phosphorus, which are vital for proper body function.
- Regulating Blood Pressure: Kidneys produce hormones like renin, which regulate blood pressure.
- **Producing Hormones**: They also produce erythropoietin, which stimulates red blood cell production, and activate vitamin D, crucial for bone health.

When kidneys are damaged, they lose the ability to perform these functions efficiently, leading to the buildup of waste and imbalances in electrolytes. The renal diet is specifically designed to address these issues.

Key Components of the Renal Diet

1. **Protein Management**
   - Purpose: Reducing protein intake can lessen the burden on the kidneys by decreasing the production of waste products like urea.
   - Sources: Lean meats, poultry, fish, and eggs in controlled portions; high-quality plant-based proteins such as beans and lentils may also be included in limited amounts.

2. **Sodium Restriction**
   - Purpose**: Lowering sodium intake helps control blood pressure and reduce fluid retention, which is crucial for kidney patients.
   - Sources: Avoid processed foods, canned soups, salty snacks, and restaurant meals. Opt for fresh or frozen vegetables, low-sodium versions of foods, and use herbs and spices for seasoning.

3. **Potassium Control**
   - Purpose: High potassium levels can cause dangerous heart rhythms, especially in individuals with compromised kidney function.
   - Sources: Limit or avoid high-potassium foods like bananas, oranges, potatoes, tomatoes, and dairy. Instead, choose lower-

potassium options such as apples, berries, grapes, and cauliflower.

4. **Phosphorus Limitation**
   - Purpose: Excess phosphorus can weaken bones and cause calcium deposits in blood vessels, eyes, lungs, and heart.
   - Sources: Restrict high-phosphorus foods like dairy products, nuts, seeds, and dark colas. Choose lower-phosphorus alternatives like rice milk, non-dairy creamers, and certain vegetables.

5. **Fluid Intake**
   - Purpose: Managing fluid intake helps prevent fluid overload, which can lead to swelling, high blood pressure, and heart issues.
   - Sources: Follow your healthcare provider's recommendations on fluid restrictions, which may include all liquids and foods that turn to liquid at room temperature (e.g., ice, soups, and gelatin).

Balancing Nutrition and Enjoyment

Adhering to a renal diet doesn't mean sacrificing flavor or enjoyment. With careful planning and creativity, you can prepare delicious meals that meet your dietary needs. Here are some strategies to maintain a balanced and enjoyable diet:

- **Use Herbs and Spices**: Enhance flavors without adding sodium by using a variety of herbs, spices, lemon juice, and vinegar.
- **Experiment with Cooking Methods**: Try baking, grilling, roasting, or steaming to bring out natural flavors in food.
- **Focus on Fresh Ingredients**: Utilize fresh fruits (low in potassium), vegetables, and lean proteins to create nutritious meals.
- **Portion Control**: Be mindful of portion sizes, especially when it comes to protein and high-potassium foods.

Working with a Dietitian

A registered dietitian specializing in renal nutrition can be an invaluable resource. They can provide personalized advice and meal plans tailored to your specific health needs, helping you navigate dietary restrictions while ensuring you receive adequate nutrition.

Common Challenges and Solutions

1. **Dining Out:** Choose restaurants that offer customizable dishes. Ask for sauces and dressings on the side, and select dishes that are steamed, grilled, or baked.
2. **Traveling:** Plan ahead by packing kidney-friendly snacks and researching restaurant menus to make informed choices.

3. **Cooking for Family:** Prepare meals that the whole family can enjoy by using renal-friendly ingredients and seasoning options that can be added at the table.

Monitoring and Adjustments

Regular monitoring of blood tests and kidney function is crucial for those on a renal diet. Your healthcare provider may adjust dietary recommendations based on changes in your condition, ensuring that your diet continues to meet your needs.

Final Thoughts

The renal diet is a crucial component of managing kidney disease, designed to reduce the workload on your kidneys while providing essential nutrients. By understanding the importance of managing protein, sodium, potassium, phosphorus, and fluid intake, and by working closely with a healthcare team, individuals can maintain their health and quality of life. Embracing this dietary approach requires commitment and creativity, but the rewards of improved well-being and kidney function are well worth the effort.

Benefits of a Renal Diet

The renal diet is specifically tailored to meet the needs of individuals with chronic kidney disease (CKD) or those undergoing dialysis. This diet plays a pivotal role in managing kidney health and overall well-being by focusing on the regulation of certain nutrients that can burden compromised kidneys. Here are the extensive benefits of adhering to a renal diet:

1. **Slows the Progression of Kidney Disease**

One of the primary benefits of a renal diet is its ability to slow the progression of kidney disease. By carefully managing the intake of proteins, sodium, potassium, and phosphorus, the renal diet reduces the workload on the kidneys. This can help preserve existing kidney function and delay the need for dialysis or transplantation.

- **Protein Management:** Reducing protein intake decreases the production of waste products like urea, which kidneys have to filter out. This reduces the strain on the kidneys.
- **Sodium Reduction:** Lowering sodium intake helps control blood pressure and reduces fluid retention, both of which are critical for kidney health.

2. **Maintains Electrolyte Balance**

The kidneys play a crucial role in maintaining the balance of electrolytes such as sodium, potassium, and phosphorus. When kidney function is compromised, these electrolytes can become imbalanced, leading to serious health issues. A renal diet helps in maintaining the balance of these critical minerals:

- **Potassium Control:** Managing potassium intake prevents

hyperkalemia, a condition characterized by dangerously high levels of potassium in the blood, which can lead to heart complications.l
- Phosphorus Limitation: Controlling phosphorus intake prevents hyperphosphatemia, which can cause bone and cardiovascular issues.

3. Reduces the Risk of Cardiovascular Disease

Cardiovascular disease is a common complication of chronic kidney disease. The renal diet helps mitigate this risk by managing blood pressure and reducing fluid retention through sodium restriction. Moreover, controlling phosphorus levels can prevent vascular calcification, where calcium deposits form in the blood vessels, contributing to heart disease.

4. Improves Nutritional Status

CKD patients often face malnutrition due to dietary restrictions and loss of appetite. A well-planned renal diet ensures that individuals receive adequate nutrition while adhering to the necessary restrictions. It includes nutrient-dense foods that provide essential vitamins and minerals without overburdening the kidneys.

- Vitamin Supplementationp: While certain foods are restricted, the renal diet often includes vitamin supplementation to ensure patients receive necessary nutrients, especially water-soluble vitamins that might be lost during dialysis.
- Balanced Meals: Emphasizing balanced meals that include a variety of low-potassium fruits and vegetables, lean proteins, and whole grains helps maintain overall health.

5. Manages Fluid Retention

Excess fluid buildup is a common problem for individuals with CKD, leading to swelling (edema), high blood pressure, and breathing difficulties. The renal diet helps manage fluid intake to prevent these issues:

- Fluid Restriction: By controlling fluid intake, the diet helps prevent fluid overload, reducing the risk of edema and heart complications.
- Sodium Control: Lowering sodium intake minimizes fluid retention, as sodium promotes water retention in the body.

6. Enhances Quality of Life

Adhering to a renal diet can significantly improve the quality of life for CKD patients. By managing symptoms and preventing complications, individuals can experience better overall health and well-being. Benefits include:

- Symptom Management: Proper dietary management can help reduce symptoms like nausea, swelling, and fatigue, which are common in CKD.
- Energy Levels: Improved nutrition and balanced electrolyte levels contribute to

higher energy levels and better physical functioning.

7. Supports Bone Health

Kidney disease often leads to imbalances in calcium and phosphorus, which can weaken bones and lead to conditions such as osteodystrophy. The renal diet helps protect bone health by:

- Phosphorus Control: Limiting high-phosphorus foods helps prevent the leaching of calcium from bones, reducing the risk of bone disease.
- Calcium Balance: Ensuring adequate but not excessive calcium intake supports bone strength and overall skeletal health.

8. Facilitates Personalized Care

A renal diet is often customized to meet the specific needs of the individual based on their stage of kidney disease, blood test results, and overall health status. This personalized approach ensures that dietary recommendations are tailored to the unique requirements of each patient, leading to better health outcomes.

- Dietitian Support: Working with a registered dietitian specializing in renal nutrition helps patients navigate dietary restrictions and ensures they receive appropriate nutrition.
- Regular Monitoring: Ongoing adjustments to the diet based on regular blood tests and kidney function assessments help maintain optimal health.

9. Prevents Dialysis Complications

For those on dialysis, a renal diet is crucial in managing the balance of fluids and electrolytes that dialysis cannot completely control. This includes:

- Minimizing Waste: By reducing the intake of certain foods, the diet helps in minimizing the waste products that dialysis needs to remove, making the process more efficient.
- Preventing Imbalances: The diet helps prevent sudden changes in electrolyte levels that can occur between dialysis sessions, reducing the risk of complications.

Essential Nutrients and Restrictions in a Renal Diet

A renal diet is meticulously designed to support kidney function and overall health by managing the intake of certain nutrients that can be taxing on the kidneys. Understanding these essential nutrients and their restrictions is crucial for individuals with chronic kidney disease (CKD) or those on dialysis. Here's an in-depth look at these key components:

1. Protein

- **Essential Role:**
  Proteins are crucial for building and repairing tissues, producing enzymes and hormones, and supporting the immune system.
- **Restriction Reasons:**
  The kidneys filter out waste products from protein metabolism, such as urea. In CKD, impaired kidney function makes it harder to remove these waste products, leading to their buildup in the blood.
- **Guidelines:**
  Early CKD: Moderate protein intake is recommended to reduce the load on the kidneys.
- Dialysis: Higher protein intake is needed to compensate for protein loss during dialysis, but it must be balanced to prevent excessive waste buildup.
- **Sources:**
  Recommended: Lean meats (chicken, turkey), fish, egg whites, low-fat dairy, and high-quality plant proteins (beans, lentils) in controlled portions.
- To Limit: Red meats, full-fat dairy, and processed meats (bacon, sausages) due to their high phosphorus and sodium content.

2. **Sodium**

- **Essential Role:**
  Sodium helps maintain fluid balance, transmit nerve signals, and support muscle function.
- **Restriction Reasons:**
  Excessive sodium intake can lead to fluid retention, high blood pressure, and swelling, exacerbating kidney problems and increasing cardiovascular risks.
- **Guidelines:**
  Limit sodium intake to 2,000 mg per day or less, as advised by a healthcare provider.
- **Sources:**
  Recommended: Fresh or frozen vegetables, fresh meats, homemade meals with no added salt, and low-sodium alternatives.
- To Avoid: Processed foods, canned soups, salty snacks, pickles, and restaurant meals. Always check labels for sodium content.

3. **Potassium**

- **Essential Role:**
  Potassium is vital for muscle function, nerve signaling, and maintaining proper heart rhythms.
- **Restriction Reasons:**
  In CKD, the kidneys' ability to excrete excess potassium is diminished, leading to hyperkalemia, a dangerous condition that can cause irregular heartbeats and muscle weakness.
- **Guidelines:**
  Monitor and limit potassium intake based on blood test results. The typical recommendation is 2,000-3,000 mg per

day, but this varies depending on individual needs.

- **Sources:**
  Recommended (Low-Potassium): Apples, berries, grapes, pineapples, cauliflower, cabbage, and white bread.

- **To Limit or Avoid (High-Potassium):** Bananas, oranges, potatoes, tomatoes, spinach, dairy products, and whole grains.

4. **Phosphorus**

- **Essential Role:**
- Phosphorus is necessary for building and maintaining bones and teeth, and it plays a role in energy production and storage.
- **Restriction Reasons:**
- CKD reduces the kidneys' ability to excrete excess phosphorus, leading to hyperphosphatemia. This can cause calcium to leach from bones, weakening them, and can lead to dangerous calcium deposits in blood vessels and organs.
- **Guidelines:**
- Limit phosphorus intake to 800-1,000 mg per day, as recommended by healthcare providers.
- **Sources:**
- Recommended (Low-Phosphorus): Fresh fruits and vegetables, rice milk, non-dairy creamers, and certain cereals.
- To Avoid (High-Phosphorus): Dairy products, nuts, seeds, beans, colas, and processed foods with added phosphorus.

5. **Fluids**

- **Essential Role:**
- Fluids are essential for digestion, absorption, circulation, and temperature regulation.
- **Restriction Reasons:**
- In CKD, especially in advanced stages or for those on dialysis, the kidneys cannot remove excess fluids efficiently, leading to fluid buildup, which can cause swelling, high blood pressure, and heart problems.
- **Guidelines:**
- Fluid intake recommendations vary based on the stage of CKD, level of kidney function, and whether the individual is on dialysis. It's typically necessary to monitor and limit all forms of fluid, including soups, ice, and gelatins.
- **Sources:**
- Recommended: Small amounts of water, controlled portions of low-potassium fruits and vegetables, and adhering strictly to healthcare providers' guidelines.
- To Manage: Track all fluid intake, including hidden sources like ice cubes, soups, and high-water-content foods.

6. **Calcium**

- **Essential Role:**
- Calcium is critical for bone health, muscle function, and nerve signaling.
- **Restriction Reasons:**
- In CKD, calcium balance can be disrupted, leading to either deficiency or excess, both of which can cause health problems. It's important to manage calcium intake in conjunction with phosphorus to avoid complications.
- **Guidelines:**

- Adjust calcium intake based on dietary restrictions and phosphorus levels. Often, calcium supplements are prescribed to ensure adequate intake without excessive phosphorus.

- **Sources:**
- Recommended: Fortified almond or rice milk, certain low-phosphorus vegetables, and calcium supplements if prescribed.
- To Limit: Dairy products (which are high in both calcium and phosphorus) and calcium supplements that also contain high phosphorus.

7. Vitamins and Minerals

- **Essential Role:**
- Vitamins and minerals support numerous body functions, including metabolism, immune response, and cellular function.
- **Restriction Reasons:**
- Certain vitamins and minerals may need to be limited or supplemented based on the individual's health status and dietary restrictions.

- **Guidelines:**
- Water-Soluble Vitamins: B vitamins and vitamin C are often supplemented as they can be lost during dialysis.
- Fat-Soluble Vitamins: Vitamins A, D, E, and K should be managed carefully to avoid toxicity, especially since vitamin D activation is impaired in CKD.
- **Sources:**
- Recommended: Specific renal multivitamins as prescribed, and a balanced diet that meets the unique needs of CKD patients.
- To Avoid: Over-the-counter supplements not specifically designed for renal patients, as they may contain inappropriate amounts of certain nutrients.

1

BREAKFAST

Low-Phosphorus Pancakes

- **Preparation Time:** 10 minutes
- **Cooking Time:** 15 minutes
- **Total Time:** 25 minutes

Ingredients

- 1 cup all-purpose flour
- 1 tablespoon sugar
- 1 teaspoon baking powder (low-phosphorus)
- 1/2 teaspoon baking soda
- 1/4 teaspoon salt
- 1 cup rice milk or almond milk (unsweetened)
- 1 large egg
- 2 tablespoons vegetable oil
- 1 teaspoon vanilla extract
- 1/2 cup fresh blueberries (optional, for added flavor and nutrition)

Procedures
1. In a large bowl, whisk together the flour, sugar, baking powder, baking soda, and salt.
2. In another bowl, combine the rice milk or almond milk, egg, vegetable oil, and vanilla extract. Beat until well mixed.
3. Gradually add the wet ingredients to the dry ingredients, stirring gently until just combined. Do not overmix; some lumps are okay.
4. Fold in the fresh blueberries if using.
5. Heat a non-stick griddle or large skillet over medium heat. Lightly grease with a small amount of vegetable oil or cooking spray.
6. Pour about 1/4 cup of batter onto the griddle for each pancake. Cook until bubbles form on the surface and the edges look set, about 2-3 minutes. Flip and cook for an additional 1-2 minutes until golden brown.
7. Serve the pancakes warm with a low-phosphorus topping such as fresh berries, a small amount of maple syrup, or a dollop of whipped cream.

Nutritional Values (per serving of 2 pancakes)
- Calories: 180
- Protein: 4g
- Carbohydrates: 28g
- Dietary Fiber: 2g
- Sugars: 6g
- Fat: 6g
- Saturated Fat: 1g
- Cholesterol: 35mg
- Sodium: 220mg
- Potassium: 60mg
- Phosphorus: 50mg

Tips for Making Low-Phosphorus Pancakes

1. **Use Low-Phosphorus Baking Powder:** Regular baking powder contains a significant amount of phosphorus. Opt for low-phosphorus or phosphorus-free baking powder available in health food stores or online.
2. **Choose the Right Milk Substitute:** Almond milk or rice milk is preferable over dairy milk as they contain significantly less phosphorus.
3. **Monitor Portion Sizes:**

Keep portion sizes moderate to help manage phosphorus intake effectively.

4. **Enhance Flavor Naturally:**

Use vanilla extract and fresh fruit to enhance flavor without adding phosphorus-rich ingredients.

5. **Check Labels:**

Always check ingredient labels for hidden phosphorus additives, especially in processed foods and baking products.

Health Benefits

- **Kidney-Friendly:**

These pancakes are tailored to be low in phosphorus, making them suitable for individuals with CKD who need to limit their phosphorus intake to prevent complications like bone and cardiovascular problems.

- **Balanced Nutrition:**

Provides a good balance of carbohydrates, protein, and fat, supporting overall energy levels and nutrient intake while adhering to renal diet restrictions.

- **Heart Health:**

Using vegetable oil instead of butter or high-saturated fat oils helps maintain heart health by providing healthier fats.

- **Customizable:**

Easily customizable with different fruits or low-phosphorus toppings to keep meals interesting and varied without compromising dietary restrictions.

- **Low Sodium:**

Controlling sodium intake helps manage blood pressure and reduce fluid retention, which is crucial for kidney health.

- **Source of Fiber:**

Adding blueberries or other fruits increases fiber content, promoting digestive health and helping to maintain stable blood sugar levels.

Herb-Infused Egg White Omelet

- **Preparation Time:** 10 minutes
- **Cooking Time:** 10 minutes
- **Total Time**: 20 minutes

Ingredients

- 4 large egg whites
- 1/4 cup diced red bell pepper
- 1/4 cup diced zucchini
- 1/4 cup diced mushrooms
- 2 tablespoons chopped fresh parsley
- 1 tablespoon chopped fresh chives
- 1 tablespoon chopped fresh basil
- 1 tablespoon olive oil (or a small amount of non-stick cooking spray)
- Salt and pepper to taste (use salt sparingly)
- Optional: a pinch of garlic powder for added flavor

Procedures

1. Dice the red bell pepper, zucchini, and mushrooms. Chop the fresh parsley, chives, and basil. Separate the egg whites from the yolks.
2. Heat a non-stick skillet over medium heat. Add the olive oil or spray lightly with non-stick cooking spray.
3. Add the diced bell pepper, zucchini, and mushrooms to the skillet. Sauté for 3-4 minutes until the vegetables are tender. Remove the vegetables from the skillet and set them aside.
4. In a bowl, whisk the egg whites until slightly frothy. Season with a small pinch of salt, pepper, and a pinch of garlic powder if desired.
5. Pour the egg whites into the skillet and cook over medium-low heat. Allow the egg whites to set without stirring, gently lifting the edges with a spatula to let uncooked egg flow underneath.
6. Once the egg whites are mostly set but still slightly runny on top, sprinkle the sautéed vegetables evenly over one half of the omelet.
7. Sprinkle the chopped parsley, chives, and basil over the vegetables.
8. Carefully fold the other half of the omelet over the filling using a spatula. Cook for another minute or until the egg whites are completely set and the omelet is heated through.
9. Slide the omelet onto a plate and serve immediately. Garnish with additional fresh herbs if desired.

Nutritional Values (per serving)

- Calories: 120
- Protein: 12g
- Carbohydrates: 4g
- Dietary Fiber: 1g
- Sugars: 2g
- Fat: 6g
- Saturated Fat: 1g
- Cholesterol: 0mg
- Sodium: 150mg
- Potassium: 250mg
- Phosphorus: 70mg

Tips for Making a Herb-Infused Egg White Omelet

- Fresh herbs add vibrant flavor and nutrients to the omelet. If fresh herbs are unavailable, dried herbs can be used, but use them sparingly as their flavor is more concentrated.
- Using a non-stick skillet helps prevent the egg whites from sticking and ensures easy flipping and folding of the omelet.
- Cook the egg whites over medium-low heat to avoid overcooking or browning. This ensures a tender and fluffy omelet.
- Experiment with different low-potassium vegetables and herbs to keep the omelet interesting and tailored to your taste preferences.
- Use salt sparingly to keep sodium levels low, which is important for kidney health. Enhance flavor with herbs and spices instead.

Health Benefits

- Egg whites are low in phosphorus, making them an excellent protein source for individuals with CKD who need to manage phosphorus intake to prevent bone and cardiovascular issues.
- Egg whites provide high-quality protein essential for tissue repair and maintenance without the extra phosphorus found in egg yolks.
- This omelet is naturally low in sodium, helping to control blood pressure and reduce fluid retention, crucial for kidney health.
- Fresh herbs like parsley, chives, and basil are rich in vitamins A, C, and K, as well as antioxidants that support overall health and immune function.
- This omelet is low in calories and fat, making it a healthy choice for weight management and cardiovascular health.
- Olive oil provides healthy monounsaturated fats that support heart health by lowering bad cholesterol levels.
- The vegetables in the omelet add dietary fiber, which promotes healthy digestion and regular bowel movements.
- Herbs and vegetables in the omelet provide antioxidants that help fight oxidative stress and inflammation, promoting overall health.

Cinnamon Quinoa Porridge

- **Preparation Time:** 5 minutes
- **Cooking Time:** 20 minutes
- **Total Time:** 25 minutes

Ingredients

- 1 cup quinoa, rinsed
- 2 cups water
- 1 cup almond milk or rice milk (unsweetened)
- 1 teaspoon ground cinnamon
- 1 tablespoon honey or maple syrup (optional)
- 1/2 teaspoon vanilla extract
- Fresh berries (blueberries, strawberries) or sliced apple for topping
- 1 tablespoon chopped nuts (such as almonds or walnuts, optional)
- Pinch of salt

Procedures

1. Rinse the quinoa thoroughly under cold water to remove its natural coating (saponin), which can cause bitterness.
2. In a medium saucepan, combine the rinsed quinoa and water. Bring to a boil over medium-high heat.
3. Once boiling, reduce the heat to low, cover, and simmer for about 15 minutes or until the water is absorbed and the quinoa is tender. Fluff with a fork.
4. Add the almond milk, ground cinnamon, and a pinch of salt to the cooked quinoa. Stir well to combine.
5. Continue to cook over low heat, stirring occasionally, until the mixture thickens to your desired consistency, about 5 minutes.
6. Stir in the honey or maple syrup (if using) and vanilla extract. Adjust the sweetness to taste.
7. Divide the quinoa porridge into bowls. Top with fresh berries or sliced apple and a sprinkle of chopped nuts if desired.

Nutritional Values (per serving, makes 2 servings)

- Calories: 250
- Protein: 6g
- Carbohydrates: 45g
- Dietary Fiber: 5g
- Sugars: 10g (with honey/maple syrup)
- Fat: 5g
- Saturated Fat: 0.5g
- Cholesterol: 0mg
- Sodium: 70mg
- Potassium: 200mg
- Phosphorus: 100mg

Tips for Making Cinnamon Quinoa Porridge

- Always rinse quinoa to remove its bitter coating. This enhances the flavor and ensures a pleasant taste.

- Opt for almond milk or rice milk instead of dairy milk to keep phosphorus levels low.
- Adjust the amount of honey or maple syrup according to your preference. You can also use stevia or another low-calorie sweetener if desired.
- Top with fresh fruits and a small amount of chopped nuts to add flavor, texture, and additional nutrients.
- Serve moderate portions to manage overall nutrient intake, especially important for those with CKD.
- Incorporate a variety of low-potassium fruits to keep the porridge nutritious and flavorful without exceeding dietary restrictions.

The fiber in quinoa also helps lower cholesterol levels.
- The combination of protein and fiber in quinoa helps regulate blood sugar levels, making it a good choice for those with diabetes or at risk of diabetes.
- Fresh berries and cinnamon add antioxidants that protect the body against oxidative stress and inflammation.
- Quinoa porridge is filling and versatile, keeping you satiated longer and reducing the likelihood of overeating.

Health Benefits

- Quinoa is lower in phosphorus and potassium compared to other grains, making it suitable for individuals with CKD.
- Quinoa is a complete protein, providing all essential amino acids. This is beneficial for maintaining muscle mass and overall health.
- The high fiber content promotes healthy digestion, helps maintain stable blood sugar levels, and supports heart health.
- Cinnamon has anti-inflammatory and antioxidant properties, which can help reduce inflammation and support overall health.
- Almond milk provides healthy fats that support cardiovascular health.

2

LIGHT AND FRESH SALAD

Cucumber Dill Salad

- **Preparation Time:** 10 minutes
- **Total Time:** 10 minutes

Ingredients

- 2 large cucumbers, thinly sliced
- 1/4 cup red onion, thinly sliced
- 2 tablespoons fresh dill, finely chopped
- 2 tablespoons lemon juice
- 2 tablespoons olive oil
- Salt and pepper to taste

Procedures

1. Wash the cucumbers thoroughly and slice them thinly. Thinly slice the red onion. Finely chop the fresh dill.
2. In a large mixing bowl, combine the sliced cucumbers, red onion, and chopped dill.
3. Drizzle the lemon juice and olive oil over the cucumber mixture.
4. Season with salt and pepper to taste.
5. Gently toss the salad until all ingredients are evenly coated with the dressing.
6. For best results, refrigerate the salad for about 30 minutes to allow the flavors to meld together before serving.
7. Serve the cucumber dill salad chilled or at room temperature as a refreshing side dish.

Nutritional Values (per serving, makes 4 servings)

- Calories: 60
- Total Fat: 5g
- Saturated Fat: 0.7g
- Cholesterol: 0mg
- Sodium: 150mg
- Total Carbohydrates: 4g
- Dietary Fiber: 1g
- Sugars: 2g
- Protein: 1g

Tips for Making Cucumber Dill Salad

- Opt for fresh cucumbers, red onions, and dill to ensure the best flavor and texture for your salad.
- Thinly sliced cucumbers absorb the flavors of the dressing better and create a more delicate texture in the salad.
- Taste the salad after adding the lemon juice, olive oil, salt, and pepper, and adjust the seasonings as needed to suit your preferences.
- Chilling the salad for a short time before serving allows the flavors to meld together and enhances the overall taste.
- Customize your cucumber dill salad by adding ingredients like cherry tomatoes, feta cheese, olives, or avocado for additional flavor and texture.

Health Benefits

- Cucumbers have a high water content, making this salad hydrating

and refreshing, especially during hot weather.
- Cucumber dill salad is low in calories but rich in vitamins, minerals, and antioxidants, making it a great option for weight management and overall health.
- Cucumbers are a good source of vitamin K, vitamin C, potassium, and various antioxidants, contributing to overall health and well-being.
- The fiber in cucumbers and onions supports digestive health by promoting regular bowel movements and preventing constipation.
- Olive oil used in the dressing provides heart-healthy monounsaturated fats, while cucumbers contain compounds that may help lower blood pressure and reduce the risk of heart disease.
- Dill possesses anti-inflammatory properties and may help reduce inflammation in the body, supporting overall health and reducing the risk of chronic diseases.
- The vitamin C from lemon juice boosts the immune system and helps the body fight off infections and illnesses.

Berry Spinach Salad with Lemon Vinaigrette

Preparation Time: 15 minutes
Total Time: 15 minutes

Ingredients

For the Salad:
- 6 cups fresh spinach leaves, washed and dried.
- 1 cup mixed berries (such as strawberries, blueberries, raspberries, and blackberries), washed and dried.
- 1/4 cup sliced almonds or chopped walnuts.
- 1/4 cup crumbled feta cheese or goat cheese (optional).
- 1/4 cup thinly sliced red onion (optional).

For the Lemon Vinaigrette:
- 1/4 cup extra virgin olive oil
- 2 tablespoons freshly squeezed lemon juice
- 1 teaspoon Dijon mustard
- 1 teaspoon honey or maple syrup
- Salt and pepper to taste

Procedures

1. Wash and dry the spinach leaves and berries. Slice the strawberries if they are large. If using, thinly slice the red onion.
2. In a small bowl, whisk together the extra virgin olive oil, lemon juice, Dijon mustard, honey or maple syrup, salt, and pepper until well combined. Set aside.
3. In a large salad bowl, combine the spinach leaves, mixed berries, sliced almonds or chopped walnuts, crumbled feta cheese or goat cheese (if using), and sliced red onion (if using).
4. Drizzle the lemon vinaigrette over the salad ingredients. Gently toss the salad until all ingredients are evenly coated with the dressing.
5. Serve the berry spinach salad immediately as a refreshing side dish or light meal.

Nutritional Values (per serving, makes 4 servings)

- Calories: 180
- Total Fat: 15g
- Saturated Fat: 2g
- Cholesterol: 5mg
- Sodium: 130mg
- Total Carbohydrates: 11g
- Dietary Fiber: 4g
- Sugars: 5g
- Protein: 4g

Tips for Making Berry Spinach Salad with Lemon Vinaigrette

- Select fresh, high-quality ingredients for the best flavor and texture. Look

- for vibrant spinach leaves and ripe, colorful berries.
- Feel free to customize the salad by adding other ingredients such as avocado, grilled chicken or tofu, cucumber, or quinoa for added protein and texture.
- Toast the sliced almonds or chopped walnuts in a dry skillet over medium heat for a few minutes until fragrant and golden brown. This adds a delicious nutty flavor to the salad.
- You can prepare the lemon vinaigrette ahead of time and store it in an airtight container in the refrigerator for up to a week. Simply shake or whisk the dressing again before using.
- If using cheese, such as feta or goat cheese, crumble or sprinkle it lightly over the salad to avoid overpowering the flavors. Alternatively, serve the cheese on the side for individual preference.

Health Benefits

- Berries are packed with antioxidants, such as vitamin C and flavonoids, which help protect cells from damage caused by free radicals and reduce the risk of chronic diseases.
- Spinach is a nutritional powerhouse, rich in vitamins A, C, and K, as well as folate, iron, and calcium, promoting overall health and well-being.
- Extra virgin olive oil in the lemon vinaigrette provides heart-healthy monounsaturated fats, which may help lower bad cholesterol levels and reduce the risk of heart disease.
- Spinach and berries are both excellent sources of dietary fiber, promoting digestive health, regulating blood sugar levels, and aiding in weight management.
- Spinach is high in vitamin K, essential for bone health and promoting proper blood clotting.
- Berries and spinach have high water content, contributing to hydration and overall well-being.
- This salad is low in calories but filling, making it a great option for weight management and maintaining a healthy lifestyle.

Zesty Quinoa and Veggie Salad

Preparation Time: 15 minutes
Total Time: 30 minutes (including quinoa cooking time)

Ingredients

For the Salad:
- 1 cup quinoa, rinsed
- 2 cups water or vegetable broth
- 1 cup cherry tomatoes, halved
- 1 cup cucumber, diced
- 1 cup bell peppers (red, yellow, or orange), diced
- 1/2 cup red onion, finely chopped
- 1/4 cup fresh parsley, chopped
- 1/4 cup fresh cilantro, chopped
- 1/4 cup black olives, sliced (optional)

For the Zesty Dressing:
- 1/4 cup extra virgin olive oil
- 2 tablespoons freshly squeezed lemon juice
- 1 clove garlic, minced
- 1 teaspoon Dijon mustard
- 1 teaspoon honey or maple syrup
- Salt and pepper to taste

Procedures

1. In a medium saucepan, combine the rinsed quinoa and water or vegetable broth. Bring to a boil over medium-high heat.
2. Once boiling, reduce the heat to low, cover, and simmer for about 15 minutes or until the quinoa is cooked and the liquid is absorbed. Fluff with a fork and let cool.
3. While the quinoa is cooking, prepare the vegetables by washing, chopping, and slicing them as indicated in the ingredients list.
4. In a small bowl, whisk together the extra virgin olive oil, lemon juice, minced garlic, Dijon mustard, honey or maple syrup, salt, and pepper until well combined. Set aside.
5. In a large mixing bowl, combine the cooked and cooled quinoa with the prepared vegetables (cherry tomatoes, cucumber, bell peppers, red onion), chopped parsley, chopped cilantro, and sliced black olives (if using).
6. Drizzle the zesty dressing over the quinoa and veggie mixture. Gently toss until all ingredients are evenly coated with the dressing.
7. For enhanced flavor, refrigerate the salad for about 30 minutes to allow the flavors to meld together before serving.
8. Serve the zesty quinoa and veggie salad chilled or at room temperature as a refreshing side dish or light meal.

Nutritional Values (per serving, makes 4 servings)

- Calories: 250
- Total Fat: 12g
- Saturated Fat: 1.5g
- Cholesterol: 0mg
- Sodium: 200mg
- Total Carbohydrates: 30g

- Dietary Fiber: 5g
- Sugars: 4g
- Protein: 6g

Tips for Making Zesty Quinoa and Veggie Salad

- Rinsing quinoa removes its bitter outer coating (saponin) and ensures a milder flavor in the salad.
- The zesty dressing adds tanginess and depth of flavor to the salad. Adjust the seasoning and sweetness according to your taste preferences.
- Feel free to customize the salad with your favorite vegetables or whatever is in season. Additional options include avocado, spinach, kale, carrots, or radishes.
- Boost the protein content of the salad by adding grilled chicken, tofu, chickpeas, or beans.
- Fresh herbs like parsley and cilantro add brightness and freshness to the salad. Don't skip them!
- You can prepare the quinoa, chop the vegetables, and make the dressing ahead of time for quick assembly when ready to serve.

Health Benefits

- Quinoa is a complete protein, containing all nine essential amino acids, making this salad a satisfying and nutritious option, especially for vegetarians and vegans.
- Quinoa and vegetables are rich in dietary fiber, promoting digestive health, regulating blood sugar levels, and keeping you feeling full and satisfied.
- The variety of vegetables in the salad provide essential vitamins (such as vitamin C, vitamin A, and vitamin K) and minerals (such as potassium and magnesium) vital for overall health and well-being.
- Extra virgin olive oil in the dressing provides heart-healthy monounsaturated fats, which may help reduce the risk of heart disease and improve cholesterol levels.
- The colorful array of vegetables in the salad provides a wide range of antioxidants, which help protect cells from damage caused by free radicals and reduce the risk of chronic diseases.
- Cucumbers and other water-rich vegetables contribute to hydration, helping to maintain proper bodily functions and overall well-being.

3

SAVORY SOUPS AND STEWS

Hearty Vegetable Soup

Preparation Time: 15 minutes
Cooking Time: 30 minutes
Total Time: 45 minutes

Ingredients

- 2 tablespoons olive oil
- 1 onion, diced
- 2 cloves garlic, minced
- 2 carrots, diced
- 2 celery stalks, diced
- 1 bell pepper (any color), diced
- 1 zucchini, diced
- 1 cup diced tomatoes (fresh or canned)
- 4 cups vegetable broth
- 2 cups water
- 1 teaspoon dried thyme
- 1 teaspoon dried oregano
- 1 bay leaf
- Salt and pepper to taste
- Fresh parsley or basil for garnish (optional)

Procedures

1. In a large pot, heat the olive oil over medium heat. Add the diced onion and cook until translucent, about 5 minutes. Add the minced garlic and cook for another minute until fragrant.
2. Add the diced carrots, celery, bell pepper, and zucchini to the pot. Cook for 5-7 minutes, stirring occasionally, until the vegetables start to soften.
3. Stir in the diced tomatoes, vegetable broth, and water. Add the dried thyme, dried oregano, and bay leaf. Season with salt and pepper to taste.
4. Bring the soup to a boil, then reduce the heat to low. Cover and simmer for 20-25 minutes, or until the vegetables are tender and flavors have melded together.
5. Taste the soup and adjust the seasoning with more salt and pepper if needed. Remove the bay leaf before serving. Ladle the soup into bowls and garnish with fresh parsley or basil if desired.

Nutritional Values (per serving, makes 4 servings)

- Calories: 150
- Total Fat: 7g
- Saturated Fat: 1g
- Cholesterol: 0mg
- Sodium: 800mg
- Total Carbohydrates: 20g
- Dietary Fiber: 5g
- Sugars: 8g
- Protein: 4g

Tips for Making Hearty Vegetable Soup

- Fresh vegetables will provide the best flavor and texture for your soup. However, canned tomatoes can be used if fresh ones are not available.
- Feel free to add or substitute vegetables based on personal preference or what you have on hand. Popular additions include potatoes, green beans, spinach, or kale.

- Dried herbs like thyme and oregano add depth of flavor to the soup. You can also experiment with other herbs and spices such as rosemary, parsley, or paprika.
- Add cooked beans, lentils, or grains like barley or quinoa to make the soup more filling and nutritious.
- This soup can be made ahead of time and stored in the refrigerator for up to 3-4 days or frozen for longer storage. Reheat gently on the stovetop or in the microwave before serving.

Health Benefits

- Hearty vegetable soup is loaded with vitamins, minerals, and antioxidants from the variety of vegetables used, promoting overall health and well-being.
- This soup is naturally low in calories and fat, making it a great option for those watching their weight or trying to maintain a healthy diet.
- The combination of vegetables and broth provides dietary fiber, which aids in digestion, promotes bowel regularity, and helps control blood sugar levels.
- Soups are an excellent way to increase fluid intake and stay hydrated, especially during colder months when water consumption may decrease.
- Vegetables like carrots, bell peppers, and tomatoes are rich in vitamins A and C, which support a healthy immune system and help protect against infections.
- The olive oil used in the soup provides heart-healthy monounsaturated fats, while the vegetables contribute to a diet rich in fiber and antioxidants, which may reduce the risk of heart disease.
- Enjoying a bowl of vegetable soup before a meal can help reduce overall calorie intake and promote satiety, potentially aiding in weight management efforts.

Chicken and Rice Soup

Preparation Time: 15 minutes
Cooking Time: 30 minutes
Total Time: 45 minutes

Ingredients

- 1 tablespoon olive oil
- 1 onion, diced
- 2 carrots, diced
- 2 celery stalks, diced
- 2 cloves garlic, minced
- 6 cups chicken broth (homemade or store-bought)
- 1 cup cooked chicken, shredded or diced
- 1 cup cooked rice (white or brown)
- 1 teaspoon dried thyme
- Salt and pepper to taste
- Fresh parsley for garnish (optional)

Procedures

1. In a large pot, heat the olive oil over medium heat. Add the diced onion, carrots, and celery. Cook for 5-7 minutes, or until the vegetables are softened.
2. Add the minced garlic and dried thyme to the pot. Cook for an additional minute, until fragrant.
3. Pour in the chicken broth, scraping up any browned bits from the bottom of the pot. Bring the soup to a simmer.
4. Stir in the cooked chicken and rice. Simmer for 10-15 minutes to allow the flavors to meld together and the soup to thicken slightly.
5. Season the soup with salt and pepper to taste. Adjust the seasoning as needed.
6. Ladle the chicken and rice soup into bowls. Garnish with fresh parsley if desired. Serve hot and enjoy!

Nutritional Values (per serving, makes 4 servings)

- Calories: 250
- Total Fat: 8g
- Saturated Fat: 2g
- Cholesterol: 35mg
- Sodium: 800mg
- Total Carbohydrates: 25g
- Dietary Fiber: 2g
- Sugars: 3g
- Protein: 18g

Tips for Making Chicken and Rice Soup

- To save time, use pre-cooked rotisserie chicken from the store. Simply shred or dice the chicken and add it to the soup during the final steps of cooking.
- Cooking the rice separately helps control the texture of the soup. Add cooked rice to the soup just before serving to prevent it from becoming mushy.
- Feel free to add other vegetables such as peas, corn, or spinach to the soup for added flavor and nutrition.
- For the best flavor, use homemade chicken broth. If using store-bought

broth, look for low-sodium options to control the saltiness of the soup.
- For a creamier texture, stir in a splash of heavy cream or coconut milk at the end of cooking.
- Fresh herbs like parsley, dill, or chives add brightness and freshness to the soup. Add them just before serving for the best flavor.

Health Benefits

- Chicken is a lean source of protein, which is essential for muscle growth and repair, as well as overall health and well-being.
- The combination of chicken, vegetables, and rice provides a wide range of essential nutrients including vitamins, minerals, and antioxidants.
- Chicken soup is not only comforting but also hydrating, helping to keep you warm and nourished during cold weather or illness.
- The vegetables and broth in chicken and rice soup provide dietary fiber, which supports digestive health and promotes regular bowel movements.
- Chicken soup has long been considered a remedy for colds and flu due to its immune-boosting properties. The combination of nutrients in the soup helps support a healthy immune system.
- Chicken and rice soup is gentle on the stomach and easy to digest, making it a suitable option for those with digestive issues or during recovery from illness.

Lentil and Sweet Potato Stew

Preparation Time: 15 minutes
Cooking Time: 45 minutes
Total Time: 1 hour

Ingredients

- 1 tablespoon olive oil
- 1 onion, diced
- 2 cloves garlic, minced
- 2 carrots, diced
- 2 celery stalks, diced
- 2 sweet potatoes, peeled and diced
- 1 cup dry lentils (green or brown), rinsed and drained
- 4 cups vegetable broth
- 1 can (14 ounces) diced tomatoes
- 1 teaspoon ground cumin
- 1 teaspoon ground coriander
- 1/2 teaspoon smoked paprika
- Salt and pepper to taste
- Fresh parsley or cilantro for garnish (optional)

Procedures

1. In a large pot or Dutch oven, heat the olive oil over medium heat. Add the diced onion and cook until softened, about 5 minutes. Add the minced garlic and cook for an additional minute until fragrant.
2. Add the diced carrots, celery, sweet potatoes, and rinsed lentils to the pot. Stir to combine with the onions and garlic.
3. Pour in the vegetable broth and add the diced tomatoes (including the juices from the can). Stir well to combine.
4. Add the ground cumin, ground coriander, smoked paprika, salt, and pepper to the pot. Stir to evenly distribute the spices. Bring the stew to a boil, then reduce the heat to low. Cover and simmer for 30-35 minutes, or until the lentils and sweet potatoes are tender.
5. Taste the stew and adjust the seasoning with salt and pepper if needed. If desired, garnish with fresh parsley or cilantro before serving.

Nutritional Values (per serving, makes 6 servings)

- Calories: 250
- Total Fat: 3g
- Saturated Fat: 0.5g
- Cholesterol: 0mg
- Sodium: 600mg
- Total Carbohydrates: 48g
- Dietary Fiber: 14g
- Sugars: 9g
- Protein: 12g

Tips for Making Lentil and Sweet Potato Stew

- Green or brown lentils hold their shape well and provide a nice texture in the stew. Avoid using red lentils, as they tend to become mushy when cooked.

- To save time, chop the vegetables and measure out the spices before starting to cook.
- Feel free to add other vegetables such as spinach, kale, or bell peppers to the stew for added flavor and nutrition.
- Add a pinch of red pepper flakes or a dash of hot sauce if you prefer a spicier stew.
- Lentil and sweet potato stew pairs well with crusty bread, rice, or quinoa for a complete and satisfying meal.
- Store any leftovers in an airtight container in the refrigerator for up to 3-4 days. Reheat gently on the stovetop or in the microwave before serving.

Health Benefits

- Lentils and sweet potatoes are both rich in dietary fiber, which supports digestive health, regulates blood sugar levels, and helps you feel full and satisfied.
- This stew is packed with vitamins, minerals, and antioxidants from the vegetables and lentils, promoting overall health and well-being.
- Lentils are an excellent source of plant-based protein, making this stew a great option for vegetarians and vegans.
- The fiber, potassium, and antioxidants in lentils and sweet potatoes support heart health by reducing cholesterol levels, lowering blood pressure, and promoting healthy blood vessels.
- The combination of fiber, protein, and complex carbohydrates in this stew helps keep you full and satisfied, making it a nutritious option for weight management.
- The vitamins, minerals, and antioxidants in the stew support a healthy immune system and help protect against infections and illnesses.

4

DELICIOUS MAIN COURSES

Herb-Crusted Baked Cod

Preparation Time: 15 minutes
Cooking Time: 20 minutes
Total Time: 35 minutes

Ingredients

- 4 cod fillets (about 6 ounces each)
- 1 cup breadcrumbs (preferably whole wheat)
- 1/4 cup grated Parmesan cheese
- 2 tablespoons fresh parsley, chopped
- 1 tablespoon fresh dill, chopped
- 1 tablespoon fresh thyme, chopped
- 2 cloves garlic, minced
- 1 lemon (zest and juice)
- 3 tablespoons olive oil
- Salt and pepper to taste
- Lemon wedges for serving (optional)

Procedures

1. Preheat your oven to 400°F (200°C). Line a baking sheet with parchment paper or lightly grease it with olive oil.
2. In a medium bowl, combine the breadcrumbs, grated Parmesan cheese, chopped parsley, chopped dill, chopped thyme, minced garlic, lemon zest, and 2 tablespoons of olive oil. Mix well to form a crumbly mixture.
3. Pat the cod fillets dry with paper towels. Season both sides with salt and pepper. Place the fillets on the prepared baking sheet.
4. Spoon the herb mixture evenly over the top of each cod fillet, pressing gently to adhere. Drizzle the remaining tablespoon of olive oil over the fillets.
5. Bake in the preheated oven for 15-20 minutes, or until the cod is cooked through and flakes easily with a fork. The internal temperature should reach 145°F (63°C).
6. Remove the cod from the oven and drizzle with fresh lemon juice. Serve immediately with lemon wedges on the side if desired.

Nutritional Values (per serving, makes 4 servings)

Calories: 300
Total Fat: 12g
Saturated Fat: 3g
Cholesterol: 70mg
Sodium: 400mg
Total Carbohydrates: 16g
Dietary Fiber: 2g
Sugars: 1g
Protein: 32g

Tips for Making Herb-Crusted Baked Cod

- Fresh herbs provide the best flavor. If fresh herbs are not available, you can substitute with dried herbs, but use half the amount as dried herbs are more concentrated.
- Feel free to add other herbs like basil, chives, or oregano based on your preference. The herb mixture can be tailored to your taste.
- For extra crunch, you can mix some crushed nuts like almonds or walnuts into the breadcrumb mixture.
- Keep an eye on the cod while baking to prevent overcooking, which can make the fish dry. Cod cooks quickly and should be just opaque and flaky.

- Serve the herb-crusted cod with a side of steamed vegetables, a fresh salad, or quinoa for a balanced meal.
- Store any leftovers in an airtight container in the refrigerator for up to 2 days. Reheat gently in the oven to maintain the crispiness of the herb crust.
- Fresh herbs and garlic in the herb crust offer antioxidant properties that help protect the body from oxidative stress and inflammation.

Health Benefits

- Cod is a high-protein, low-fat fish, making it an excellent choice for those looking to increase their protein intake while keeping calories low.
- Cod is a good source of omega-3 fatty acids, which are beneficial for heart health, reducing inflammation, and supporting brain function.
- This dish is relatively low in calories, making it suitable for weight management and those on calorie-restricted diets.
- Cod is rich in essential vitamins and minerals such as vitamin B12, iodine, and selenium, which support various bodily functions, including metabolism, thyroid function, and immune health.
- The combination of healthy fats from olive oil and omega-3 fatty acids from the cod can help lower cholesterol levels and reduce the risk of heart disease.
- The addition of Parmesan cheese provides calcium, which is important for maintaining strong bones and teeth.

Grilled Lemon Chicken

Marinating Time: 30 minutes to 2 hours
Preparation Time: 10 minutes
Cooking Time: 15-20 minutes
Total Time: 55 minutes to 2 hours and 30 minutes

Ingredients

- 4 boneless, skinless chicken breasts
- 1/4 cup olive oil
- 1/4 cup freshly squeezed lemon juice (about 2 lemons)
- Zest of 1 lemon
- 3 cloves garlic, minced
- 1 tablespoon fresh thyme, chopped
- 1 tablespoon fresh rosemary, chopped
- 1 teaspoon salt
- 1/2 teaspoon black pepper
- Lemon wedges for serving (optional)
- Fresh parsley for garnish (optional)

Procedures

1. In a small bowl, whisk together the olive oil, lemon juice, lemon zest, minced garlic, chopped thyme, chopped rosemary, salt, and black pepper
2. Place the chicken breasts in a resealable plastic bag or a shallow dish. Pour the marinade over the chicken, ensuring each piece is well-coated. Seal the bag or cover the dish and refrigerate for at least 30 minutes, preferably up to 2 hours for maximum flavor.
3. Preheat your grill to medium-high heat (about 400°F/200°C). If using a charcoal grill, prepare a two-zone fire.
4. Remove the chicken from the marinade and let the excess drip off. Place the chicken breasts on the preheated grill. Grill for 6-8 minutes per side, or until the internal temperature reaches 165°F (75°C) and the chicken is cooked through. Avoid moving the chicken too much to get nice grill marks.
5. Transfer the grilled chicken to a plate and let it rest for 5 minutes before serving. This allows the juices to redistribute, ensuring moist and tender chicken. Serve with lemon wedges and garnish with fresh parsley if desired.

Nutritional Values (per serving, makes 4 servings)

- Calories: 300
- Total Fat: 14g
- Saturated Fat: 2g
- Cholesterol: 90mg
- Sodium: 500mg
- Total Carbohydrates: 2g
- Dietary Fiber: 0g
- Sugars: 0g
- Protein: 38g

Tips for Making Grilled Lemon Chicken

- Fresh lemon juice and zest, along with fresh herbs, provide the best flavor. Avoid using bottled lemon juice or dried herbs if possible.
- While 30 minutes is sufficient for marinating, allowing the chicken to marinate for up to 2 hours will infuse it with more flavor. Do not marinate for longer than 4 hours as the acidity of the lemon can start to break down the chicken fibers, making it mushy.
- Pound the chicken breasts to an even thickness to ensure they cook evenly on the grill. This also helps to tenderize the chicken.
- Brush the grill grates with oil or use a grill spray to prevent the chicken from sticking. This also helps achieve those desirable grill marks.
- Use a meat thermometer to check the internal temperature of the chicken. It should reach 165°F (75°C) to be safe for consumption. Overcooking can make the chicken dry.
- Serve grilled lemon chicken with a side of steamed vegetables, a fresh salad, or quinoa for a balanced meal. It also pairs well with a light, citrusy vinaigrette.

Health Benefits

- Chicken breasts are an excellent source of lean protein, which is essential for muscle growth and repair, as well as overall health.
- This dish is relatively low in calories, making it suitable for weight management and those on calorie-restricted diets.
- Chicken provides essential vitamins and minerals such as B vitamins, phosphorus, and selenium, which support energy production, bone health, and immune function.
- Olive oil, used in the marinade, is rich in monounsaturated fats, which are beneficial for heart health. These fats can help reduce bad cholesterol levels and lower the risk of heart disease.
- Fresh herbs like thyme and rosemary contain antioxidants that help protect the body from oxidative stress and inflammation.
- The vitamin C from the lemon juice helps boost the immune system, supports skin health, and aids in the absorption of iron from the chicken.
- The garlic in the marinade not only adds flavor but also has prebiotic properties, which promote healthy digestion by supporting the growth of beneficial gut bacteria.

Vegetarian Stuffed Peppers

Preparation Time: 20 minutes
Cooking Time: 45 minutes
Total Time: 1 hour 5 minutes

Ingredients

- 4 large bell peppers (any color)
- 1 cup cooked quinoa (or rice, bulgur, or couscous)
- 1 tablespoon olive oil
- 1 onion, diced
- 2 cloves garlic, minced
- 1 zucchini, diced
- 1 carrot, grated
- 1 (14 oz) can ,Mmatoes
- 1 (15 oz) can black beans, drained and rinsed
- 1 cup corn kernels (fresh, frozen, or canned)
- 1 teaspoon ground cumin
- 1 teaspoon smoked paprika
- 1/2 teaspoon chili powder
- Salt and pepper to taste
- 1 cup shredded mozzarella or cheddar cheese (optional)
- Fresh cilantro or parsley for garnish (optional)

Procedures

1. Preheat your oven to 375°F (190°C). Cut the tops off the bell peppers and remove the seeds and membranes. If needed, trim the bottoms slightly to help them stand upright. Place the peppers in a baking dish.
2. Heat the olive oil in a large skillet over medium heat. Add the diced onion and cook until softened, about 5 minutes. Add the minced garlic and cook for another minute until fragrant.
3. Stir in the diced zucchini and grated carrot. Cook for about 5 minutes, until the vegetables are tender. Add the diced tomatoes, black beans, and corn. Stir in the ground cumin, smoked paprika, chili powder, salt, and pepper. Cook for another 5 minutes, allowing the flavors to meld.
4. Stir the cooked quinoa into the vegetable mixture until well combined. Taste and adjust seasoning if necessary.
5. Spoon the filling mixture into the prepared bell peppers, packing it down gently. If using, sprinkle the shredded cheese on top of each stuffed pepper.
6. Cover the baking dish with foil and bake in the preheated oven for 30 minutes. Remove the foil and bake for an additional 15 minutes, or until the peppers are tender and the cheese (if used) is melted and bubbly.
7. Remove from the oven and let cool slightly before serving. Garnish with fresh cilantro or parsley if desired. Enjoy hot.

Nutritional Values (per serving, makes 4 servings)

- Calories: 350
- Total Fat: 10g
- Saturated Fat: 2g
- Cholesterol: 10mg
- Sodium: 600mg
- Total Carbohydrates: 55g
- Dietary Fiber: 14g
- Sugars: 10g
- Protein: 12g

Tips for Making Vegetarian Stuffed Peppers

- Use large, firm bell peppers that can stand upright and have enough space for filling. A variety of colors can make the dish more visually appealing.
- Feel free to customize the filling based on your preferences. You can add other vegetables like mushrooms, spinach, or chopped kale. For added protein, consider incorporating lentils or tofu.
- To make this dish vegan, simply omit the cheese or use a plant-based cheese alternative.
- For even softer peppers, you can precook them by boiling them for 5 minutes before stuffing. This step is optional but can be helpful if you prefer very tender peppers.
- Fresh herbs like basil, oregano, or thyme can enhance the flavor of the filling. Adjust the spices to your taste preference for a more customized dish.
- Stuffed peppers can be prepared ahead of time and stored in the refrigerator for up to 2 days before baking. Leftovers can be stored in an airtight container for up to 3 days and reheated in the oven or microwave.

Health Benefits

- The combination of vegetables, beans, and grains in this dish provides a substantial amount of dietary fiber, which aids digestion and promotes satiety.
- Bell peppers are an excellent source of vitamins A and C, which support immune function, skin health, and vision. The vegetables and beans add additional vitamins and minerals, including potassium, folate, and iron.
- Black beans and quinoa provide plant-based protein, essential for muscle repair and maintenance, making this dish a great option for vegetarians and vegans.
- The colorful vegetables and spices in this dish are rich in antioxidants, which help protect the body from oxidative stress and inflammation.
- This dish is low in calories and high in fiber, making it a filling and satisfying meal that can support weight management efforts.
- The ingredients in vegetarian stuffed peppers contribute to heart health by providing dietary fiber, healthy fats from olive oil, and plant-based nutrients that can help lower cholesterol levels and reduce the risk of heart disease.
- The high fiber content helps regulate blood sugar levels by slowing the absorption of sugar into the

bloodstream, making it a good option for individuals managing diabetes or blood sugar concerns.

Garlic and Herb Pork Tenderloin

Marinating Time: 30 minutes to 2 hours (optional but recommended)
Preparation Time: 15 minutes
Cooking Time: 25-30 minutes
Total Time: 1 hour 10 minutes to 2 hours 45 minutes

Ingredients

- 2 pork tenderloins (about 1 pound each)
- 4 cloves garlic, minced
- 2 tablespoons fresh rosemary, finely chopped
- 2 tablespoons fresh thyme, finely chopped
- 1 tablespoon fresh parsley, finely chopped
- 1 teaspoon dried oregano
- 1 teaspoon salt
- 1/2 teaspoon black pepper
- 3 tablespoons olive oil
- 1 tablespoon lemon juice
- 1 teaspoon lemon zest

Procedures

1. In a small bowl, combine the minced garlic, chopped rosemary, thyme, parsley, dried oregano, salt, pepper, olive oil, lemon juice, and lemon zest. Mix well to form a paste.
2. Pat the pork tenderloins dry with paper towels. Rub the garlic and herb mixture all over the tenderloins, ensuring they are well-coated. Place the tenderloins in a resealable plastic bag or a shallow dish, cover, and refrigerate for at least 30 minutes and up to 2 hours. This step is optional but allows the flavors to penetrate the meat.
3. Preheat your oven to 400°F (200°C). If you have an oven-safe skillet, it will make the transition from stovetop to oven easier.
4. Heat 1 tablespoon of olive oil in a large oven-safe skillet over medium-high heat. Once hot, add the pork tenderloins and sear on all sides until golden brown, about 2-3 minutes per side. This helps to lock in the juices and add flavor.
5. Transfer the skillet to the preheated oven. Roast the pork for 15-20 minutes, or until the internal temperature reaches 145°F (63°C) for medium-rare or 160°F (71°C) for medium. Use a meat thermometer to ensure accuracy.
6. Remove the pork from the oven and transfer to a cutting board. Let it rest for 5-10 minutes before slicing. This allows the juices to redistribute throughout the meat, ensuring it remains tender and juicy.
7. Slice the pork tenderloin into 1/2-inch thick slices. Serve immediately with your choice of sides, such as roasted vegetables, mashed potatoes, or a fresh salad.

Nutritional Values (per serving, makes 6 servings)

- Calories: 220

- Total Fat: 11g
- Saturated Fat: 2g
- Cholesterol: 80mg
- Sodium: 450mg
- Total Carbohydrates: 1g
- Dietary Fiber: 0g
- Sugars: 0g
- Protein: 28g

Tips for Making Garlic and Herb Pork Tenderloin

- Ensure to trim any silver skin from the pork tenderloin before marinating. Silver skin is a tough, silvery membrane that can make the meat chewy if not removed.
- Pork tenderloin is a lean cut of meat that can dry out quickly if overcooked. Use a meat thermometer to check for doneness and remove from the oven as soon as it reaches the desired internal temperature.
- Allowing the pork to rest after cooking is crucial for retaining its juices. Cutting into the meat too soon can cause the juices to run out, resulting in a drier dish.
- Fresh herbs provide the best flavor for this dish. If fresh herbs are not available, dried herbs can be used, but use about half the amount as they are more concentrated.
- You can marinate the pork tenderloin up to 24 hours in advance. The longer marinating time will enhance the flavors even more.
- Pair the pork tenderloin with a variety of side dishes such as roasted vegetables, garlic mashed potatoes, or a simple green salad to complement the flavors.

Health Benefits

- Pork tenderloin is an excellent source of lean protein, which is essential for muscle growth, repair, and overall body function.
- This cut of pork is relatively low in fat, making it a healthier option compared to other fattier cuts of meat.
- Pork provides essential nutrients such as B vitamins (B6 and B12), zinc, and selenium, which are important for energy metabolism, immune function, and overall health.
- The fresh herbs used in the marinade, such as rosemary, thyme, and parsley, contain antioxidants that help protect the body from oxidative stress and inflammation.
- Olive oil, a key ingredient in the marinade, is rich in monounsaturated fats, which can help lower bad cholesterol levels and reduce the risk of heart disease.
- Garlic has natural antibacterial and antiviral properties, which can help boost the immune system and promote overall health.
- Herbs and garlic not only add flavor but also have digestive health benefits, promoting better digestion and nutrient absorption.

Zucchini Noodles with Pesto

Preparation Time: 20 minutes
Cooking Time: 5 minutes
Total Time: 25 minutes

Ingredients

For the Zucchini Noodles:
- 4 medium zucchini, spiralized
- 1 tablespoon olive oil
- Salt and pepper to taste

For the Pesto:
- 2 cups fresh basil leaves, packed
- 1/2 cup grated Parmesan cheese
- 1/2 cup pine nuts (can substitute with walnuts or almonds)
- 2 cloves garlic
- 1/2 cup extra virgin olive oil
- Salt and pepper to taste
- 1 tablespoon lemon juice (optional)

Procedures

1. Use a spiralizer to turn the zucchini into noodles (zoodles). If you don't have a spiralizer, you can use a julienne peeler or a mandoline slicer to create thin strips resembling noodles.
2. In a food processor, combine the basil leaves, Parmesan cheese, pine nuts, and garlic. Pulse until the ingredients are finely chopped.
3. With the processor running, slowly drizzle in the extra virgin olive oil until the mixture is smooth and well combined. If you prefer a thinner consistency, add a bit more olive oil.
4. Season with salt and pepper to taste. Add lemon juice if using, and pulse once more to combine.
5. Heat 1 tablespoon of olive oil in a large skillet over medium-high heat. Add the zucchini noodles and sauté for 2-3 minutes until they are just tender but still have some crunch. Do not overcook, as zucchini noodles can become watery and mushy.
6. Season with a pinch of salt and pepper.
7. Remove the skillet from the heat and add the pesto to the zucchini noodles. Toss to coat the noodles evenly with the pesto sauce.
8. Serve immediately, garnished with additional Parmesan cheese and fresh basil leaves if desired.

Nutritional Values (per serving, makes 4 servings)

- Calories: 350
- Total Fat: 32g
- Saturated Fat: 6g
- Cholesterol: 10mg
- Sodium: 350mg
- Total Carbohydrates: 10g
- Dietary Fiber: 3g
- Sugars: 5g
- Protein: 8g

Tips for Making Zucchini Noodles with Pesto

- Fresh basil and high-quality olive oil are key to making a vibrant and flavorful pesto. Avoid using dried basil as it won't provide the same fresh taste.
- To prevent zucchini noodles from becoming too watery, lightly salt them and let them sit for about 10 minutes before cooking. This helps to draw out excess moisture. Pat them dry with a paper towel before sautéing.
- Zucchini noodles are best served immediately after cooking. If they sit too long, they can release water and become soggy.
- Feel free to customize your pesto by adding other herbs like parsley or cilantro, or by using different nuts such as walnuts or almonds.
- A food processor works best for making a smooth and well-blended pesto. However, you can also use a blender or a mortar and pestle for a more rustic texture.
- For a more complete meal, consider adding grilled chicken, shrimp, or tofu to the dish.
- Store any leftover pesto in an airtight container in the refrigerator for up to a week. You can also freeze pesto in ice cube trays for longer storage. Zucchini noodles are best eaten fresh but can be stored in the refrigerator for a day or two.

- Zucchini noodles are a great low-calorie and low-carb alternative to traditional pasta, making them suitable for weight management and low-carb diets.
- Zucchini is rich in vitamins A, C, and K, as well as potassium and fiber. These nutrients support immune function, skin health, and cardiovascular health.
- The olive oil in the pesto provides healthy monounsaturated fats that can help reduce bad cholesterol levels and lower the risk of heart disease.
- Basil, a key ingredient in pesto, is high in antioxidants which help protect the body from oxidative stress and inflammation.
- Zucchini contains fiber that aids in digestion and helps maintain a healthy gut. The fiber also promotes satiety, helping you feel full for longer.
- Garlic, used in the pesto, has natural antibacterial and antiviral properties that can help boost the immune system and fight off infections.
- Parmesan cheese is a good source of calcium and phosphorus, both of which are essential for maintaining strong bones and teeth.

Health Benefits

5

SATISFYING SIDES

Roasted Brussels Sprouts with Lemon

Preparation Time: 10 minutes
Cooking Time: 25-30 minutes
Total Time: 35-40 minutes

Ingredients

- 1 1/2 pounds Brussels sprouts
- 2 tablespoons olive oil
- 1 teaspoon salt
- 1/2 teaspoon black pepper
- 1 lemon (zest and juice)
- 2 cloves garlic, minced
- 1/4 cup grated Parmesan cheese (optional)
- Fresh parsley, chopped (for garnish, optional)

Procedures

1. Preheat your oven to 400°F (200°C). Line a baking sheet with parchment paper or lightly grease it with olive oil.
2. Trim the ends of the Brussels sprouts and remove any yellow or damaged outer leaves. Cut the sprouts in half lengthwise. If they are particularly large, you can quarter them to ensure even roasting.
3. In a large bowl, toss the Brussels sprouts with olive oil, salt, and black pepper. Make sure they are evenly coated.
4. Spread the Brussels sprouts in a single layer on the prepared baking sheet, cut side down. This helps them to caramelize and become crispy.
5. Roast in the preheated oven for 20-25 minutes, until they are golden brown and tender. Shake the pan or stir the sprouts halfway through the cooking time to ensure even roasting.
6. While the sprouts are roasting, zest and juice the lemon. Mince the garlic.
7. In the last 5 minutes of roasting, sprinkle the minced garlic over the Brussels sprouts. This allows the garlic to cook slightly without burning.
8. Remove the sprouts from the oven and immediately toss them with the lemon zest and lemon juice.
9. Transfer the roasted Brussels sprouts to a serving dish. If using, sprinkle with grated Parmesan cheese and fresh parsley. Serve hot.

Nutritional Values (per serving, makes 4 servings)

- Calories: 120
- Total Fat: 7g
- Saturated Fat: 1g
- Cholesterol: 0mg
- Sodium: 600mg
- Total Carbohydrates: 12g
- Dietary Fiber: 5g
- Sugars: 3g
- Protein: 4g

Tips for Making Roasted Brussels Sprouts with Lemon

- Look for fresh, firm Brussels sprouts with tight, bright green leaves. Avoid those with yellowing leaves or a strong odor.
- Cut the Brussels sprouts to a uniform size to ensure even cooking. Larger sprouts should be halved or quartered.
- Spread the sprouts out in a single layer on the baking sheet without overcrowding. Overcrowding can cause the sprouts to steam instead of roast, leading to less caramelization.
- Adding garlic in the last few minutes of roasting prevents it from burning and turning bitter, while still allowing it to cook and release its flavor.
- Adding lemon zest and juice right after roasting adds a bright, fresh flavor that complements the nuttiness of the roasted sprouts.
- Grated Parmesan cheese adds a savory, umami flavor that pairs well with the Brussels sprouts and lemon. It can be omitted for a vegan option.
- Adjust the amount of salt, pepper, and lemon juice to suit your taste preferences. Fresh herbs like parsley or thyme can also be added for extra flavor.

Health Benefits

- Brussels sprouts are a powerhouse of nutrients, including vitamins C and K, folate, and manganese. They are also high in fiber, which aids in digestion and promotes satiety.
- Brussels sprouts contain antioxidants such as kaempferol, which help protect the body from oxidative stress and reduce inflammation.
- The high vitamin C content in Brussels sprouts boosts the immune system and enhances skin health by promoting collagen production.
- The fiber, antioxidants, and anti-inflammatory compounds in Brussels sprouts contribute to heart health by helping to lower cholesterol levels and reducing the risk of heart disease.
- Vitamin K in Brussels sprouts plays a crucial role in bone health by helping with calcium absorption and bone formation.
- Low in calories but high in fiber, Brussels sprouts are a great addition to a weight management diet. They help you feel full longer, reducing the likelihood of overeating.
- The cruciferous family of vegetables, which includes Brussels sprouts, contains glucosinolates and other compounds that may help protect against certain types of cancer.
- The fiber content aids in digestive health by promoting regular bowel movements and supporting a healthy gut microbiome.

Garlic Mashed Cauliflower

Preparation Time: 10 minutes
Cooking Time: 15-20 minutes
Total Time: 25-30 minutes

Ingredients

- 1 large head cauliflower, cut into florets
- 3 cloves garlic, minced
- 2 tablespoons butter or olive oil (for a vegan option)
- 1/4 cup grated Parmesan cheese (optional for added flavor)
- 1/4 cup milk or unsweetened almond milk (for a vegan option)
- Salt and pepper to taste
- Fresh chives or parsley, chopped (for garnish, optional)

Procedures

Wash and cut the cauliflower into florets. Discard the leaves and core.

Bring a large pot of salted water to a boil. Add the cauliflower florets and cook for about 10-15 minutes, or until the cauliflower is very tender and easily pierced with a fork. Alternatively, you can steam the cauliflower florets until they are soft and tender.

Drain the cooked cauliflower well and let it sit in the colander for a few minutes to allow excess moisture to evaporate. This step is important to prevent the mashed cauliflower from becoming too watery.

In a small skillet, heat the butter or olive oil over medium heat. Add the minced garlic and sauté until fragrant and lightly golden, about 1-2 minutes. Be careful not to burn the garlic.

Transfer the drained cauliflower to a food processor or a large mixing bowl. Add the sautéed garlic, Parmesan cheese (if using), and milk or almond milk.

Process or blend until smooth and creamy. If you prefer a chunkier texture, use a potato masher or an immersion blender to mash the cauliflower to your desired consistency.

Season with salt and pepper to taste. Transfer the mashed cauliflower to a serving bowl and garnish with chopped fresh chives or parsley, if desired.

Serve immediately as a side dish.

Nutritional Values (per serving, makes 4 servings)

- Calories: 100
- Total Fat: 5g
- Saturated Fat: 2g
- Cholesterol: 10mg
- Sodium: 200mg
- Total Carbohydrates: 10g
- Dietary Fiber: 4g
- Sugars: 3g
- Protein: 4g

Tips for Making Garlic Mashed Cauliflower

- Select a firm, white cauliflower with tight florets and minimal blemishes. Fresh cauliflower ensures a better texture and flavor.
- After cooking, ensure the cauliflower is well-drained and let it sit to evaporate excess moisture. This step

helps achieve a creamy consistency without being watery.
- For a super smooth texture, use a food processor or high-speed blender. For a chunkier mash, a potato masher or immersion blender works well.
- If the mash is too thick, add a little more milk or almond milk until you reach the desired consistency. If it's too thin, let it sit for a few minutes to thicken up.
- Parmesan cheese adds a rich, savory flavor, but you can also use cream cheese or Greek yogurt for extra creaminess. For a vegan option, nutritional yeast can be used.
- Fresh herbs like chives, parsley, or thyme add a burst of flavor and color. Stir them in just before serving or use as a garnish.
- Garlic mashed cauliflower is best served hot. If you need to reheat it, do so gently on the stovetop or in the microwave, stirring occasionally.

Health Benefits

- Cauliflower is a great low-carb alternative to potatoes, making it suitable for low-carb and ketogenic diets. It helps in reducing overall carbohydrate intake without sacrificing flavor or satisfaction.
- Cauliflower is rich in dietary fiber, which aids in digestion, promotes regular bowel movements, and helps maintain a healthy gut.
- Cauliflower provides essential vitamins and minerals such as vitamin C, vitamin K, folate, and potassium, which support overall health and well-being.
- Cauliflower contains antioxidants like vitamin C and other phytonutrients that help protect the body from oxidative stress and inflammation.
- Being low in calories and high in fiber, cauliflower helps you feel full longer, which can aid in weight management and prevent overeating.
- The fiber, antioxidants, and anti-inflammatory compounds in cauliflower contribute to heart health by helping to lower cholesterol levels and reducing the risk of heart disease.
- Vitamin K in cauliflower plays a crucial role in bone health by aiding in calcium absorption and bone formation.
- The high vitamin C content boosts the immune system, enhances skin health, and supports the body's ability to fight off infections.

Spicy Roasted Carrots

Preparation Time: 10 minutes
Cooking Time: 25-30 minutes
Total Time: 35-40 minutes

Ingredients

- 1 1/2 pounds carrots, peeled and cut into sticks or rounds
- 2 tablespoons olive oil
- 1 teaspoon ground cumin
- 1 teaspoon paprika
- 1/2 teaspoon chili powder
- 1/4 teaspoon cayenne pepper (adjust to taste)
- 1/2 teaspoon garlic powder
- Salt and pepper to taste
- 1 tablespoon honey or maple syrup (optional for added sweetness)
- Fresh cilantro or parsley, chopped (for garnish, optional)
- Lemon or lime wedges (for serving, optional)

Procedures

Preheat your oven to 425°F (220°C). Line a baking sheet with parchment paper or lightly grease it with olive oil.
Peel the carrots and cut them into uniform sticks or rounds. This ensures even cooking. If the carrots are small, you can simply halve them lengthwise.
In a large mixing bowl, combine the olive oil, ground cumin, paprika, chili powder, cayenne pepper, garlic powder, salt, and pepper. Mix well.
Add the carrots to the bowl and toss to coat them evenly with the spice mixture. If using, drizzle with honey or maple syrup and toss again to coat.
Spread the seasoned carrots in a single layer on the prepared baking sheet. Make sure they are not overlapping, to allow for even roasting and caramelization.
Roast in the preheated oven for 25-30 minutes, or until the carrots are tender and slightly caramelized, stirring or flipping them halfway through the cooking time to ensure even browning.
Remove the carrots from the oven and transfer them to a serving dish. Garnish with fresh chopped cilantro or parsley if desired.
Serve with lemon or lime wedges on the side for an extra burst of freshness.

Nutritional Values (per serving, makes 4 servings)

- Calories: 150
- Total Fat: 7g
- Saturated Fat: 1g
- Cholesterol: 0mg
- Sodium: 250mg
- Total Carbohydrates: 20g
- Dietary Fiber: 5g
- Sugar: 10g
- Protein: 2g

Tips for Making Spicy Roasted Carrots

- Cut the carrots into uniform pieces to ensure they cook evenly. Smaller pieces will roast more quickly, while larger pieces will take longer to become tender.
- Adjust the amount of cayenne pepper based on your heat preference. You can start with a smaller amount and add more if you prefer a spicier dish.
- Adding honey or maple syrup is optional but can help balance the heat from the spices with a touch of sweetness. This step is especially good if serving the carrots to children or those who prefer milder flavors.
- Spread the carrots out in a single layer on the baking sheet. Overcrowding can cause them to steam instead of roast, resulting in less caramelization and flavor.
- Fresh spices have a more robust flavor. Make sure your spices are not stale to get the best taste.
- Fresh cilantro or parsley adds a fresh, herbaceous note that complements the spicy carrots well.
- Serving with lemon or lime wedges adds a bright, tangy contrast to the spicy and sweet flavors, enhancing the overall taste.

Health Benefits

- Carrots are an excellent source of vitamins A, C, and K, potassium, and dietary fiber. Vitamin A, in the form of beta-carotene, supports eye health, immune function, and skin health.
- The spices used, such as cumin, paprika, and cayenne pepper, contain compounds with anti-inflammatory properties that can help reduce inflammation in the body.
- Carrots and spices like paprika and cumin are rich in antioxidants, which help protect the body from oxidative stress and may reduce the risk of chronic diseases.
- The dietary fiber in carrots aids in digestion, helps maintain regular bowel movements, and supports a healthy gut microbiome.
- The fiber, potassium, and antioxidants in carrots contribute to heart health by helping to lower blood pressure, reduce cholesterol levels, and prevent cardiovascular disease.
- Carrots are low in calories but high in fiber, making them a filling and nutritious option for those looking to manage their weight.
- The vitamins and antioxidants in carrots support the immune system, helping the body to fend off infections and illnesses.
- The fiber in carrots helps to slow the absorption of sugar, which can help regulate blood sugar levels and prevent spikes.

Quinoa Pilaf with Herbs

Preparation Time: 10 minutes
Cooking Time: 20-25 minutes
Total Time: 30-35 minutes

Ingredients

- 1 cup quinoa, rinsed
- 2 cups low-sodium vegetable broth or water
- 2 tablespoons olive oil
- 1 small onion, finely chopped
- 2 cloves garlic, minced
- 1 carrot, finely diced
- 1 celery stalk, finely diced
- 1/2 teaspoon salt
- 1/4 teaspoon black pepper
- 1/2 cup fresh parsley, chopped
- 1/4 cup fresh dill, chopped
- 1/4 cup fresh mint, chopped
- Zest of 1 lemon
- Juice of 1/2 lemon

Procedures

1. Place the quinoa in a fine-mesh strainer and rinse under cold water for about 2 minutes. This helps remove the natural saponins on the surface of the quinoa, which can impart a bitter taste.
2. In a medium saucepan, bring the vegetable broth or water to a boil. Add the rinsed quinoa, reduce the heat to low, cover, and simmer for about 15 minutes, or until the liquid is absorbed and the quinoa is tender. Remove from heat and let it sit, covered, for 5 minutes. Fluff with a fork.
3. While the quinoa is cooking, heat the olive oil in a large skillet over medium heat. Add the chopped onion, carrot, and celery, and sauté for about 5-7 minutes, until the vegetables are softened.
4. Add the minced garlic to the skillet and sauté for another 1-2 minutes until fragrant. Season with salt and pepper.
5. Add the cooked quinoa to the skillet with the sautéed vegetables. Stir to combine and cook for another 2-3 minutes, allowing the flavors to meld together.
6. Remove the skillet from the heat. Stir in the chopped parsley, dill, mint, lemon zest, and lemon juice. Mix well to combine all the flavors.
7. Transfer the quinoa pilaf to a serving dish and garnish with additional fresh herbs if desired. Serve warm or at room temperature.

Nutritional Values (per serving, makes 4 servings)

Calories: 200
Total Fat: 7g
- Saturated Fat: 1g
- Cholesterol: 0mg
- Sodium: 250mg
- Total Carbohydrates: 30g
- Dietary Fiber: 5g
- Sugars: 3g
- Protein: 6g

Tips for Making Quinoa Pilaf with Herbs

- Always rinse quinoa before cooking to remove the bitter-tasting saponins on its surface.
- Fresh herbs provide the best flavor. If you need to use dried herbs, use about one-third the amount called for fresh herbs.
- Feel free to add other vegetables such as bell peppers, peas, or spinach for added nutrition and flavor.
- Cooking quinoa in vegetable broth instead of water adds more depth and flavor to the dish.
- Adding lemon zest and juice at the end brightens up the flavors and adds a refreshing tang.
- Allow the quinoa to sit for a few minutes after cooking to absorb any remaining moisture and become fluffier
- Garnish with toasted nuts or seeds for added crunch and nutrition.

Health Benefits

- Quinoa is one of the few plant foods that contain all nine essential amino acids, making it a complete protein source. This is particularly beneficial for vegetarians and vegans.
- Quinoa is high in dietary fiber, which aids in digestion, promotes regular bowel movements, and helps maintain a healthy weight.
- Naturally gluten-free, quinoa is a great option for those with celiac disease or gluten intolerance.
- Quinoa is rich in vitamins B and E, as well as minerals like magnesium, iron, and potassium, which are essential for overall health and well-being.
- The fresh herbs, particularly parsley, dill, and mint, are rich in antioxidants that help combat oxidative stress and inflammation in the body.
- The fiber and antioxidants in quinoa and herbs contribute to heart health by helping to lower cholesterol levels and reduce the risk of heart disease.
- The fiber in quinoa helps regulate blood sugar levels by slowing the absorption of sugar into the bloodstream, making it a good choice for those managing diabetes.
- High fiber content supports healthy digestion and a balanced gut microbiome, which is crucial for overall health.
- Quinoa is low in calories but high in protein and fiber, making it a filling and nutritious option for those looking to manage their weight.

6

SNACK TIME

Baked Kale Chips

Preparation Time: 10 minutes
Cooking Time: 20 minutes
Total Time: 30 minutes

Ingredients

- 1 large bunch of kale
- 1-2 tablespoons olive oil
- 1/2 teaspoon sea salt
- Optional seasonings: garlic powder, onion powder, smoked paprika, nutritional yeast, or chili powder

Procedures

1. Preheat your oven to 300°F (150°C). Line a large baking sheet with parchment paper or a silicone baking mat.
2. Wash and thoroughly dry the kale. It's important to dry the kale completely to ensure it becomes crispy when baked.
3. Remove the thick stems and tough center ribs from the kale leaves. Tear the leaves into bite-sized pieces.
4. Place the kale pieces in a large bowl. Drizzle with olive oil and sprinkle with sea salt. Toss to coat the leaves evenly.
5. For added flavor, you can sprinkle on your choice of optional seasonings such as garlic powder, onion powder, smoked paprika, nutritional yeast, or chili powder. Toss again to distribute the seasonings evenly.
6. Spread the seasoned kale pieces in a single layer on the prepared baking sheet. Avoid overlapping the pieces to ensure even baking.
7. Bake in the preheated oven for 20 minutes, or until the kale is crispy and slightly browned around the edges. Keep an eye on the kale towards the end of the baking time to prevent burning.
8. Remove the baking sheet from the oven and let the kale chips cool on the sheet for a few minutes. This helps them crisp up further.
9. Transfer the kale chips to a serving bowl and enjoy immediately.

Nutritional Values (per serving, makes 4 servings)

- Calories: 70
- Total Fat: 4g
- Saturated Fat: 0.5g
- Cholesterol: 0mg
- Sodium: 150mg
- Total Carbohydrates: 7g
- Dietary Fiber: 2g
- Sugars: 1g
- Protein: 2g

Tips for Making Baked Kale Chips

- Ensure the kale is completely dry before baking. Any moisture will cause the chips to steam and become soggy instead of crispy.
- Use just enough oil to lightly coat the kale. Too much oil can make the chips greasy, while too little oil can prevent them from becoming crispy.
- Spread the kale pieces in a single layer on the baking sheet. Overlapping pieces will result in uneven baking and less crispy chips.
- Oven temperatures can vary, so keep a close eye on the kale chips, especially in the last few minutes of

baking. They can go from perfectly crispy to burnt quickly.
- Customize your kale chips with a variety of seasonings to suit your taste. Nutritional yeast adds a cheesy flavor, while smoked paprika gives a smoky depth.
- Let the kale chips cool on the baking sheet for a few minutes after baking. This helps them become even crispier.
- Store any leftover kale chips in an airtight container at room temperature for up to 2 days. However, they are best enjoyed fresh.

Health Benefits

- Kale is a nutrient-dense superfood, providing vitamins A, C, K, and B6, as well as minerals such as calcium, potassium, and magnesium. These nutrients support overall health, including immune function, bone health, and blood clotting.
- Kale chips are low in calories, making them a great snack option for those looking to manage their weight while still enjoying a satisfying treat.
- Kale is rich in antioxidants like beta-carotene, vitamin C, and various flavonoids and polyphenols. These compounds help combat oxidative stress and may reduce the risk of chronic diseases.
- The fiber, potassium, and antioxidants in kale contribute to heart health by helping to lower blood pressure, reduce cholesterol levels, and prevent cardiovascular disease.
- Kale contains compounds that have anti-inflammatory effects, which can help reduce inflammation in the body and support overall health.
- The fiber content in kale aids in digestion, promotes regular bowel movements, and supports a healthy gut microbiome.
- The high vitamin C content in kale boosts the immune system, helping the body to fight off infections and illnesses.
- Kale is a good source of calcium and vitamin K, both of which are essential for maintaining strong bones and preventing osteoporosis.

Spicy Chickpea Snack

Preparation Time: 10 minutes
Cooking Time: 40-45 minutes
Total Time: 50-55 minutes

Ingredients

- 2 cups cooked chickpeas (or 1 can, drained and rinsed)
- 2 tablespoons olive oil
- 1 teaspoon smoked paprika
- 1/2 teaspoon ground cumin
- 1/2 teaspoon chili powder
- 1/4 teaspoon cayenne pepper (adjust to taste)
- 1/2 teaspoon garlic powder
- 1/4 teaspoon salt
- 1/4 teaspoon black pepper

Procedures

- Preheat your oven to 400°F (200°C). Line a baking sheet with parchment paper or a silicone baking mat.
- If using canned chickpeas, drain and rinse them well. Pat them dry with a paper towel to remove as much moisture as possible. This helps the chickpeas become crispy when baked.
- In a large bowl, combine the olive oil, smoked paprika, ground cumin, chili powder, cayenne pepper, garlic powder, salt, and black pepper. Mix well to create a spice blend.
- Add the dried chickpeas to the bowl and toss them until they are evenly coated with the spice blend.
- Spread the seasoned chickpeas in a single layer on the prepared baking sheet. Avoid overcrowding the chickpeas to ensure even baking.
- Bake in the preheated oven for 40-45 minutes, stirring or shaking the pan every 10-15 minutes to ensure they cook evenly and become crispy. The chickpeas are done when they are golden brown and crunchy.
- Remove the baking sheet from the oven and let the chickpeas cool completely. This will help them to crisp up further.
- Once cooled, transfer the chickpeas to an airtight container. They can be stored at room temperature for up to a week.

Nutritional Values (per serving, makes 4 servings)

- Calories: 150
- Total Fat: 7g
- Saturated Fat: 1g
- Cholesterol: 0mg
- Sodium: 300mg
- Total Carbohydrates: 18g
- Dietary Fiber: 6g
- Sugars: 1g
- Protein: 6g

Tips for Making Spicy Chickpea Snack

- Removing as much moisture as possible from the chickpeas before baking is crucial for achieving a

crispy texture. Pat them dry with paper towels or a clean kitchen towel.
- Fresh, high-quality spices will yield the best flavor. Ensure your spices are not stale to enhance the taste of the snack.
- Adjust the amount of cayenne pepper to suit your heat preference. You can also experiment with other spices like curry powder, turmeric, or coriander for different flavor profiles.
- Stirring or shaking the baking sheet every 10-15 minutes during baking ensures that the chickpeas cook evenly and do not burn.
- Chickpeas should be golden brown and crispy when done. If they are still soft, continue baking them in 5-minute intervals, checking frequently to avoid burning.
- Store the chickpeas in an airtight container at room temperature. Ensure they are completely cooled before storing to maintain their crispiness.

Health Benefits

- Chickpeas are a great plant-based protein source, making them an excellent snack for vegetarians and vegans. Protein is essential for muscle repair, growth, and overall body function.
- The high fiber content in chickpeas aids in digestion, promotes regular bowel movements, and helps maintain a healthy weight by keeping you full longer.
- Chickpeas contain significant amounts of soluble fiber, which can help lower cholesterol levels. They also have a low glycemic index, which supports stable blood sugar levels.
- Chickpeas are rich in vitamins and minerals, including folate, iron, magnesium, phosphorus, and B vitamins, all of which are essential for maintaining good health and preventing nutrient deficiencies.
- The spices used in this recipe, particularly cumin and chili powder, have anti-inflammatory properties that can help reduce inflammation in the body and support overall health.
- Spices like paprika and garlic powder are rich in antioxidants, which help protect the body from oxidative stress and may reduce the risk of chronic diseases.
- Low in calories but high in protein and fiber, spicy chickpea snacks are a filling and nutritious option for those looking to manage their weight.
- The fiber in chickpeas helps regulate blood sugar levels by slowing the absorption of sugar into the bloodstream, making them a good choice for people with diabetes or those at risk of developing diabetes.
- Chickpeas promote a healthy gut by serving as a prebiotic, encouraging the growth of beneficial bacteria in the digestive tract.

Apple Slices with Almond Butter

Preparation Time: 5 minutes
Cooking Time: None
Total Time: 5 minutes

Ingredients

- 1 large apple (any variety, such as Fuji, Gala, or Granny Smith)
- 2 tablespoons almond butter
- Optional toppings: a sprinkle of cinnamon, a drizzle of honey, chia seeds, or sliced almonds

Procedures

1. Wash the apple thoroughly under running water to remove any dirt or wax.
2. Core the apple and slice it into thin wedges. You can leave the skin on for added fiber and nutrients.
3. If the almond butter is too thick, you can warm it slightly in the microwave for about 10-15 seconds to make it more spreadable. Stir well to ensure it is smooth and creamy.
4. Arrange the apple slices on a plate. Spread a small amount of almond butter on each slice. You can use a knife or a small spoon to do this.
5. If desired, add optional toppings such as a sprinkle of cinnamon, a drizzle of honey, chia seeds, or sliced almonds to enhance the flavor and texture.
6. Serve the apple slices with almond butter immediately to enjoy the crispness of the apples and the creamy texture of the almond butter.

Nutritional Values (per serving, makes 1 serving)

- Calories: 200
- Total Fat: 12g
- Saturated Fat: 1g
- Cholesterol: 0mg
- Sodium: 2mg
- Total Carbohydrates: 24g
- Dietary Fiber: 5g
- Sugars: 16g
- Protein: 4g

Tips for Making Apple Slices with Almond Butter

- Select fresh, crisp apples for the best texture and flavor. Varieties like Fuji, Gala, Honeycrisp, or Granny Smith are excellent choices.
- Use smooth almond butter for easy spreading. If using natural almond butter that has separated, stir it well to combine the oils and solids before spreading.
- If you are preparing the apple slices ahead of time, you can prevent browning by dipping them in a mixture of water and lemon juice (1 tablespoon of lemon juice per cup of water) and then patting them dry.
- Experiment with different toppings to add variety and extra nutrition. Cinnamon adds a warm, sweet flavor,

while chia seeds and sliced almonds add crunch and additional nutrients.

- For a portable snack, pack the apple slices and almond butter separately and assemble them just before eating to maintain the freshness and texture of the apples.

Health Benefits

- Apples are a great source of dietary fiber, which aids in digestion, promotes regular bowel movements, and helps maintain a healthy weight by keeping you full longer.
- Apples provide essential vitamins such as vitamin C, which boosts the immune system, and potassium, which supports heart health.
- Apples contain antioxidants like quercetin and flavonoids that help combat oxidative stress and reduce the risk of chronic diseases.
- The fiber and polyphenols in apples are linked to improved heart health by helping to lower cholesterol levels and reduce the risk of cardiovascular disease.
- Almond butter is rich in healthy fats, protein, and fiber, which provide sustained energy and help stabilize blood sugar levels.
- Almond butter is packed with nutrients, including vitamin E, magnesium, and healthy monounsaturated fats, which are beneficial for overall health.
- The protein content in almond butter supports muscle repair and growth, making this snack a good option for post-workout recovery.
- Almonds are a good source of calcium and phosphorus, which are essential for maintaining strong and healthy bones.
- The combination of fiber from the apples and protein and healthy fats from the almond butter helps keep you full and satisfied, which can aid in weight management.

7

SMOOTHIES AND BEVERAGES

Green Detox Smoothie

Preparation Time: 10 minutes
Cooking Time: None
Total Time: 10 minutes

Ingredients

- 1 cup fresh spinach leaves
- 1/2 cup kale leaves, stems removed
- 1/2 cucumber, chopped
- 1 small green apple, cored and chopped
- 1/2 ripe banana
- 1/2 lemon, juiced
- 1 tablespoon fresh ginger, peeled and chopped
- 1 tablespoon chia seeds (optional)
- 1 cup coconut water or filtered water
- Ice cubes (optional, for a colder smoothie)

Procedures

1. Wash all the fresh produce thoroughly.
2. Remove the stems from the kale and chop the cucumber and apple into smaller pieces for easier blending.
3. Peel and chop the fresh ginger.
4. In a high-speed blender, add the spinach, kale, cucumber, apple, banana, lemon juice, and fresh ginger.
5. If using, add the chia seeds for an extra boost of omega-3 fatty acids and fiber.
6. Pour in the coconut water or filtered water to facilitate blending. Add ice cubes if you prefer a colder smoothie.
7. Blend on high until all the ingredients are thoroughly combined and the smoothie is smooth and creamy. This usually takes about 1-2 minutes, depending on the power of your blender.
8. If the smoothie is too thick, add more water or coconut water a little at a time until you reach your desired consistency.
9. If it is too thin, add a few more pieces of banana or some ice cubes and blend again.
10. Pour the green detox smoothie into a glass and enjoy immediately. For an added touch, you can garnish with a slice of lemon or a few extra chia seeds.

Nutritional Values (per serving, makes 2 servings)

- Calories: 120
- Total Fat: 2g
- Saturated Fat: 0g
- Cholesterol: 0mg
- Sodium: 45mg
- Total Carbohydrates: 28g
- Dietary Fiber: 7g
- Sugars: 14g
- Protein: 3g

Tips for Making a Green Detox Smoothie

- Fresh, organic ingredients are best for maximum nutrient content and flavor.

- Ensure your greens are crisp and your fruits are ripe.
- To achieve a smooth consistency, use a high-speed blender. Blend the greens and liquids first before adding the fruits and other ingredients for a smoother texture.
- The sweetness of the banana and apple balances the bitterness of the greens. Adjust the amounts of these fruits to suit your taste preference.
- Add superfoods like spirulina, chlorella, or matcha powder for additional detoxifying benefits. You can also include a scoop of protein powder to make the smoothie more filling.
- Adding chia seeds provides extra fiber, protein, and omega-3 fatty acids. Soak them in water for a few minutes before blending to help them expand and blend more smoothly.
- While coconut water adds a subtle sweetness and electrolytes, you can also use almond milk, cashew milk, or plain water depending on your preference.

Health Benefits

- The combination of spinach, kale, cucumber, and apple provides a wide range of vitamins and minerals, including vitamins A, C, K, and several B vitamins, as well as calcium, magnesium, and potassium.
- Green vegetables and fruits are loaded with antioxidants that help protect the body from oxidative stress and reduce inflammation.
- Ingredients like spinach, kale, and cucumber are known for their detoxifying properties, helping to cleanse the liver and support the body's natural detox processes.
- The high vitamin C content from the lemon and apple boosts the immune system, helping the body fight off infections and illnesses.
- The fiber content from the fruits and vegetables aids in digestion, promotes regular bowel movements, and supports a healthy gut microbiome.
- Coconut water is rich in electrolytes, which help keep the body hydrated. Proper hydration is essential for overall health and efficient detoxification.
- Low in calories but high in nutrients and fiber, this smoothie helps keep you full and satisfied, making it a great addition to a weight management plan.
- Fresh ginger is known for its anti-inflammatory properties, which can help reduce inflammation and improve overall health.
- The natural sugars from the fruits provide a quick energy boost, while the fiber ensures a slow release of energy, preventing spikes and crashes.

Berry Banana Smoothie

Preparation Time: 5 minutes
Cooking Time: None
Total Time: 5 minutes

Ingredients

- 1 banana (ripe)
- 1 cup mixed berries (fresh or frozen; strawberries, blueberries, raspberries, and blackberries)
- 1/2 cup Greek yogurt (optional for added creaminess and protein)
- 1 cup almond milk (or any milk of your choice)
- 1 tablespoon chia seeds (optional)
- 1 tablespoon honey or maple syrup (optional, for added sweetness)
- 1/2 teaspoon vanilla extract (optional)
- Ice cubes (optional, for a thicker consistency)

Procedures

1. Peel the banana and break it into chunks.
2. If using fresh berries, rinse them under cold water. If using frozen berries, no need to thaw.
3. Measure out the Greek yogurt, almond milk, chia seeds, honey or maple syrup, and vanilla extract if using.
4. In a high-speed blender, combine the banana chunks, mixed berries, Greek yogurt, almond milk, chia seeds, honey or maple syrup, and vanilla extract.
5. Add a handful of ice cubes if you prefer a thicker, colder smoothie.
6. Blend on high for about 1-2 minutes or until the mixture is completely smooth and creamy. Scrape down the sides of the blender as needed to ensure all ingredients are well incorporated.
7. If the smoothie is too thick, add a little more almond milk and blend again until you reach your desired consistency.
8. If it's too thin, add more banana or berries and blend again.
9. Pour the smoothie into a glass and enjoy immediately. You can also garnish with a few fresh berries or a sprinkle of chia seeds for an extra touch.

Nutritional Values (per serving, makes 2 servings)

- Calories: 150
- Total Fat: 3g
- Saturated Fat: 0.5g
- Cholesterol: 5mg (if using Greek yogurt)
- Sodium: 40mg
- Total Carbohydrates: 30g
- Dietary Fiber: 6g
- Sugars: 18g
- Protein: 4g

Tips for Making a Berry Banana Smoothie

- Frozen berries make the smoothie cold and thick without needing to add ice, which can dilute the flavor.
- Use a ripe banana for natural sweetness and a smoother texture.
- Adding Greek yogurt not only makes the smoothie creamier but also increases the protein content, making it more filling.
- If the berries are tart, you may want to add a sweetener like honey or maple syrup. Taste the smoothie before adding any sweeteners to adjust according to your preference.
- Add a tablespoon of chia seeds, flax seeds, or a scoop of protein powder for an extra nutritional boost.
- Start by blending the liquids and yogurt first to create a smooth base before adding the fruits and other ingredients.
- For a fresh-tasting smoothie, consume it immediately after blending. If you need to store it, keep it in the refrigerator and consume within 24 hours.

Health Benefits

- Berries are packed with antioxidants, which help fight oxidative stress and reduce inflammation in the body.
- Both berries and bananas are excellent sources of dietary fiber, which aids in digestion, promotes regular bowel movements, and helps maintain a healthy weight.
- The vitamins and antioxidants in berries and bananas help strengthen the immune system, protecting the body against illnesses and infections.
- Berries are known for their heart-healthy benefits, including reducing blood pressure, lowering cholesterol levels, and improving overall cardiovascular health.
- The natural sugars from the fruits provide a quick energy boost, making this smoothie an excellent choice for breakfast or a pre-workout snack.
- The vitamins and antioxidants in berries can help improve skin health, promoting a glowing and youthful appearance.
- The fiber and protein in this smoothie help keep you full and satisfied, reducing the likelihood of overeating and aiding in weight management.
- Greek yogurt adds calcium and protein, both essential for maintaining strong and healthy bones.
- The high water content in fruits and the addition of almond milk or another liquid helps keep the body hydrated.
- The fiber content from the fruits supports a healthy digestive system, promoting gut health and preventing constipation.

Herbal Iced Tea

Preparation Time: 10 minutes
Cooking Time: 15 minutes
Cooling Time: 1 hour (or until chilled)
Total Time: 1 hour 25 minutes

Ingredients

- 4 cups water
- 4-5 tablespoons dried herbs or 4-5 herbal tea bags (such as chamomile, peppermint, hibiscus, rooibos, or a blend)
- 1-2 tablespoons honey, agave syrup, or your preferred sweetener (optional)
- 1-2 tablespoons fresh lemon juice (optional)
- Ice cubes
- Fresh mint leaves, lemon slices, or berries for garnish (optional)

Procedures

1. In a medium-sized pot, bring 4 cups of water to a rolling boil.
2. Once the water is boiling, remove the pot from the heat.
3. Add the dried herbs or herbal tea bags to the hot water. Cover the pot and let the herbs steep for 10-15 minutes, depending on the desired strength. The longer the steeping time, the stronger the flavor.
4. After steeping, strain the tea to remove the herbs or tea bags. Pour the tea into a large pitcher.
5. If desired, add honey, agave syrup, or your preferred sweetener while the tea is still warm. Stir well until the sweetener is completely dissolved.
6. Add fresh lemon juice to enhance the flavor and add a touch of citrus brightness.
7. Let the tea cool to room temperature, then refrigerate for at least 1 hour or until thoroughly chilled.
8. Fill glasses with ice cubes and pour the chilled herbal tea over the ice.
9. Garnish with fresh mint leaves, lemon slices, or berries if desired.
10. Serve immediately and enjoy the refreshing, flavorful taste of herbal iced tea.

Nutritional Values (per serving, makes 4 servings)

- Calories: 5 (without sweeteners)
- Total Fat: 0g
- Saturated Fat: 0g
- Cholesterol: 0mg
- Sodium: 10mg
- Total Carbohydrates: 1g
- Dietary Fiber: 0g
- Sugars: 0g (more if sweeteners are added)
- Protein: 0g

Tips for Making Herbal Iced Tea

- Use high-quality, organic dried herbs or herbal tea bags to ensure the best flavor and health benefits.

- Mix and match different herbs to create unique flavor combinations.

- Popular herbs for iced tea include chamomile, peppermint, hibiscus, lemon balm, and rooibos.
- Adjust the sweetness to your liking. You can use natural sweeteners like honey or agave syrup, or leave it unsweetened for a purely herbal taste.
- Fresh lemon juice, lime juice, or orange slices can enhance the flavor of your herbal iced tea. Adding a few sprigs of fresh herbs like mint or basil can also add a refreshing twist.
- For a sparkling version, mix the chilled herbal tea with carbonated water or soda water before serving.
- Prepare a large batch of herbal iced tea and keep it in the refrigerator for a ready-to-drink, refreshing beverage. It can typically be stored for up to 3-5 days.
- To avoid diluting the flavor, freeze some of the brewed herbal tea in ice cube trays and use these ice cubes in your iced tea.

Health Benefits

- Herbal iced tea is a delicious way to stay hydrated, especially for those who prefer a flavorful alternative to plain water.
- Many herbs used in iced tea, such as hibiscus and rooibos, are rich in antioxidants that help protect the body from oxidative stress and reduce inflammation.
- Herbs like peppermint and chamomile can help soothe digestive issues, relieve bloating, and support overall digestive health.
- Herbal teas are naturally caffeine-free, making them an excellent choice for those who are sensitive to caffeine or prefer to avoid it.
- Chamomile and lemon balm are known for their calming and relaxing properties, which can help reduce stress and promote better sleep.
- Herbs like elderberry and echinacea are often used to support the immune system and help ward off colds and infections.
- Many herbs have anti-inflammatory properties that can help reduce inflammation in the body, contributing to overall health and wellness.
- Hibiscus tea is known for its potential to lower blood pressure and support heart health.
- Antioxidants and anti-inflammatory compounds in herbal teas can contribute to healthier skin by reducing inflammation and supporting detoxification.

8

HEAITHY DESSERTS

Baked Apple with Cinnamon

Preparation Time: 10 minutes
Cooking Time: 30-40 minutes
Total Time: 40-50 minutes

Ingredients

- 4 medium-sized apples (Granny Smith, Honeycrisp, or Fuji work well)
- 1/4 cup brown sugar or coconut sugar
- 1 teaspoon ground cinnamon
- 1/4 teaspoon ground nutmeg (optional)
- 1/4 cup chopped nuts (such as walnuts or pecans, optional)
- 1/4 cup raisins or dried cranberries (optional)
- 1/4 cup rolled oats (optional, for a crumb topping)
- 2 tablespoons melted butter or coconut oil
- 1/2 cup apple juice or water

Procedures

- Preheat your oven to 350°F (175°C).
- Wash and core the apples, leaving the bottoms intact to hold the filling. Use an apple corer or a small knife to remove the core and seeds. If desired, you can peel a strip of skin from around the top of each apple to prevent them from splitting as they bake.
- In a small bowl, combine the brown sugar, ground cinnamon, and ground nutmeg. If using, add the chopped nuts, raisins or dried cranberries, and rolled oats. Mix well to combine.
- Place the prepared apples in a baking dish. Spoon the filling mixture into the hollowed-out cores of the apples, pressing down gently to pack it in. Drizzle the melted butter or coconut oil over the top of each apple.
- Pour the apple juice or water into the bottom of the baking dish. This will help keep the apples moist and prevent them from drying out during baking.
- Cover the baking dish with aluminum foil and bake in the preheated oven for 20 minutes. Remove the foil and continue baking for another 10-20 minutes, or until the apples are tender when pierced with a fork and the filling is bubbly.
- Carefully remove the baking dish from the oven. Let the apples cool for a few minutes before serving. They can be enjoyed on their own or topped with a scoop of vanilla ice cream, a dollop of whipped cream, or a drizzle of caramel sauce.

Nutritional Values (per serving, makes 4 servings)

- Calories: 180
- Total Fat: 6g
- Saturated Fat: 3g
- Cholesterol: 10mg
- Sodium: 20mg
- Total Carbohydrates: 34g
- Dietary Fiber: 5g
- Sugars: 25g

- Protein: 1g

Tips for Making Baked Apples with Cinnamon

- Select firm, tart apples like Granny Smith, Honeycrisp, or Fuji. These varieties hold their shape well during baking and provide a nice balance to the sweet filling.
- Feel free to get creative with the filling. You can add ingredients like chopped dried fruits, different nuts, or even a splash of vanilla extract for extra flavor.
- Peeling a small strip of skin around the top of each apple helps prevent the skin from splitting as the apples bake.
- Adjust the amount of sugar according to your taste preference. If you prefer a less sweet dessert, reduce the sugar or use a natural sweetener like honey or maple syrup.
- Adding a splash of lemon juice to the filling can help enhance the flavor and balance the sweetness.
- For an extra indulgent treat, serve the baked apples with a scoop of vanilla ice cream, a dollop of Greek yogurt, or a drizzle of caramel sauce.

Health Benefits

- Apples are an excellent source of dietary fiber, which aids in digestion, promotes regular bowel movements, and helps maintain a healthy weight.
- Apples are rich in vitamins such as vitamin C, which boosts the immune system, and potassium, which helps regulate blood pressure.
- Apples contain various antioxidants, including quercetin, which help protect the body from oxidative stress and reduce the risk of chronic diseases.
- The fiber, potassium, and antioxidants in apples contribute to heart health by lowering cholesterol levels and reducing the risk of cardiovascular diseases.
- The fiber in apples helps regulate blood sugar levels by slowing the absorption of sugar, making them a good choice for people with diabetes.
- The combination of fiber and the prebiotic effects of apples supports a healthy gut microbiome, promoting better digestion and overall gut health.
- The small amount of calcium and other minerals in apples can contribute to maintaining strong bones.
- Baked apples are a low-calorie dessert option that satisfies sweet cravings without the excess calories found in many traditional desserts.

Vanilla Chia Seed Pudding

Preparation Time: 10 minutes
Cooking Time: None
Chilling Time: 4 hours (or overnight)
Total Time: 4 hours 10 minutes

Ingredients

- 1/4 cup chia seeds
- 1 cup unsweetened almond milk (or any milk of your choice)
- 1 teaspoon vanilla extract
- 1-2 tablespoons maple syrup or honey (optional, for sweetness)
- Fresh fruits, nuts, seeds, or granola for topping (optional)

Procedures

1. In a medium-sized mixing bowl, combine the chia seeds, almond milk, vanilla extract, and maple syrup or honey (if using). Stir well to ensure the chia seeds are evenly distributed and not clumped together.
2. Let the mixture sit for about 5-10 minutes, then give it another good stir. This helps to prevent the chia seeds from settling at the bottom and ensures they begin to gel properly.
3. Cover the bowl with plastic wrap or transfer the mixture to an airtight container. Place it in the refrigerator and let it chill for at least 4 hours or overnight. This allows the chia seeds to absorb the liquid and form a pudding-like consistency.
4. Before serving, give the pudding a good stir to break up any clumps and ensure a smooth texture.
5. Spoon the pudding into individual serving bowls or glasses. Top with your choice of fresh fruits, nuts, seeds, or granola for added flavor and texture.
6. Serve immediately and enjoy your creamy, nutritious vanilla chia seed pudding.

Nutritional Values (per serving, makes 2 servings)

- Calories: 150
- Total Fat: 8g
- Saturated Fa: 1g
- Cholesterol: 0mg
- Sodium: 100mg
- Total Carbohydrates: 18gDietary Fiber: 10g
- Sugars: 8g
- Protein: 4g

Tips for Making Vanilla Chia Seed Pudding

- Ensure your chia seeds are fresh and not expired. Fresh seeds absorb liquid better and create a smoother pudding.
- Taste the mixture before chilling and adjust the sweetness to your preference. You can use more or less maple syrup or honey as desired.
- Different types of milk (such as coconut milk, oat milk, or dairy milk)

can be used to create different flavors and textures.

- For a smoother pudding, you can blend the mixture in a blender before chilling. This creates a more uniform and creamy consistency.
- Experiment with additional flavors by adding cocoa powder, matcha powder, or a pinch of cinnamon to the mixture before chilling.
- For a visually appealing dessert, layer the chia seed pudding with fruit purees, yogurt, or granola in a glass.

Health Benefits

- Chia seeds are an excellent source of dietary fiber, which aids in digestion, promotes regular bowel movements, and helps maintain a healthy weight.
- Chia seeds are one of the best plant-based sources of omega-3 fatty acids, which are essential for heart health and reducing inflammation.
- Chia seeds provide a good amount of plant-based protein, which is important for muscle repair and growth.
- Chia seeds contain antioxidants that help protect the body from oxidative stress and reduce the risk of chronic diseases.
- Chia seeds are rich in calcium, magnesium, and phosphorus, which are essential for maintaining strong and healthy bones.
- The fiber in chia seeds helps regulate blood sugar levels by slowing the absorption of sugar into the bloodstream, making this pudding a good choice for people with diabetes.
- Chia seeds can absorb up to 10 times their weight in water, helping to keep you hydrated and feeling full for longer.
- The combination of fiber and protein in chia seeds helps promote satiety and reduces the likelihood of overeating, supporting weight management.
- The high fiber content supports a healthy digestive system and promotes a healthy gut microbiome.

Rice Pudding with Nutmeg

Preparation Time: 10 minutes
Cooking Time: 30-40 minutes
Total Time: 40-50 minutes

Ingredients

- 1/2 cup white rice (long-grain or short-grain)
- 4 cups whole milk
- 1/2 cup granulated sugar
- 1 teaspoon vanilla extract
- 1/2 teaspoon ground nutmeg
- Pinch of salt
- 1/4 cup raisins (optional)
- Ground cinnamon for garnish (optional)

Procedures

1. Rinse the rice under cold water to remove any excess starch. Drain well.
2. In a large saucepan, combine the rinsed rice, whole milk, sugar, vanilla extract, ground nutmeg, and a pinch of salt. Stir well to combine.
3. Place the saucepan over medium heat and bring the mixture to a gentle boil, stirring frequently to prevent the rice from sticking to the bottom of the pan.
4. Once the mixture comes to a boil, reduce the heat to low and let it simmer gently, uncovered, stirring occasionally, for about 30-40 minutes or until the rice is tender and the pudding has thickened to your desired consistency. Be careful not to let it boil over.
5. If using raisins, stir them into the pudding during the last 5-10 minutes of cooking.
6. Remove the saucepan from the heat and let the pudding cool slightly before serving. You can enjoy it warm or chilled, depending on your preference.
7. Sprinkle ground cinnamon on top of the pudding just before serving for extra flavor and a decorative touch.
8. Serve the rice pudding with nutmeg as a delicious dessert or snack. Enjoy its creamy texture and comforting flavor!

Nutritional Values (per serving, makes 4 servings)

- Calories: 300
- Total Fat: 5g
- Saturated Fat: 3g
- Cholesterol: 20mg
- Sodium: 100mg
- Total Carbohydrates: 55g
- Dietary Fiber: 1g
- Sugars: 30g
- Protein: 8g

Tips for Making Rice Pudding with Nutmeg

- Use long-grain or short-grain white rice for the best texture in your pudding. Avoid using quick-cooking or instant rice, as they can become mushy.

- Stir the pudding frequently while it's cooking to prevent the rice from sticking to the bottom of the pan and ensure even cooking.
- Taste the pudding as it cooks and adjust the sweetness to your liking by adding more or less sugar.
- Feel free to experiment with different spices to flavor your rice pudding. Besides nutmeg, you can try cinnamon, cardamom, or cloves for a unique twist.
- Customize your pudding by adding chopped nuts, shredded coconut, or diced fruits like apples or pears for extra texture and flavor.
- Drizzle caramel sauce, chocolate sauce, or fruit compote over the rice pudding just before serving for an extra indulgent treat.
- Rice pudding can be made ahead of time and stored in the refrigerator for up to 3-4 days. Simply reheat it gently on the stovetop or in the microwave before serving.

Health Benefits

- Whole milk is a rich source of calcium, which is essential for maintaining strong bones and teeth.
- Rice pudding provides a good source of carbohydrates, which are the body's primary source of energy.
- Milk and rice both contain protein, which is important for muscle repair and growth.
- Rice pudding with nutmeg is a comforting and satisfying dessert that can help lift your mood and satisfy your sweet cravings.
- The fiber content in rice pudding can help support digestive health and promote regular bowel movements.
- Nutmeg contains compounds that may aid in the absorption of nutrients and promote overall gut health.
- Some studies suggest that nutmeg may have heart-protective properties and help lower cholesterol levels.

Berry Sorbet

Preparation Time: 10 minutes
Freezing Time: 4-6 hours (or overnight)
Total Time: 4 hours 10 minutes to 6 hours 10 minutes

Ingredients

- 4 cups mixed berries (such as strawberries, blueberries, raspberries, blackberries)
- 1/2 cup granulated sugar or sweetener of choice (adjust to taste)
- 2 tablespoons freshly squeezed lemon juice
- 1/4 cup water

Procedures

1. Wash the mixed berries under cold water and pat them dry with a clean kitchen towel. Remove any stems or leaves from the strawberries if necessary.
2. In a blender or food processor, combine the mixed berries, granulated sugar or sweetener of choice, freshly squeezed lemon juice, and water. Blend until smooth and well combined. If the mixture is too thick, you can add a splash of water to help it blend more easily.
3. If you prefer a smoother sorbet, you can strain the berry mixture through a fine-mesh sieve to remove any seeds or pulp. Use a spatula to press the mixture through the sieve into a bowl, leaving behind any solids.
4. Transfer the strained or unstrained berry mixture into a shallow dish or baking pan. Cover with plastic wrap or a lid and place it in the refrigerator to chill for about 1-2 hours, or until thoroughly chilled.
5. Once the mixture is chilled, pour it into the bowl of an ice cream maker and churn according to the manufacturer's instructions until it reaches a smooth and creamy consistency. Alternatively, if you don't have an ice cream maker, you can pour the mixture into a shallow dish and place it in the freezer.
6. If using the freezer method, remove the dish from the freezer every 30-45 minutes and stir the mixture vigorously with a fork to break up any ice crystals. Repeat this process several times until the sorbet is uniformly frozen and has a smooth texture.
7. Once the sorbet has reached the desired consistency, scoop it into serving bowls or glasses. Garnish with fresh berries or mint leaves if desired.
8. Serve the berry sorbet immediately and enjoy its refreshing and fruity flavor!

Nutritional Values (per serving, makes 4 servings)

- Calories: 120
- Total Fat: 0g
- Saturated Fat: 0g
- Cholesterol: 0mg
- Sodium: 0mg

- Total Carbohydrates: 30g
- Dietary Fiber: 5g
- Sugars: 20g
- Protein: 1g

Tips for Making Berry Sorbet

- You can use either fresh or frozen berries to make sorbet. If using frozen berries, there's no need to thaw them before blending.
- Taste the berry mixture before freezing and adjust the sweetness level according to your preference. You can add more or less sugar or sweetener as desired.
- Feel free to customize your sorbet by adding other fruits, such as mangoes, peaches, or pineapple, to the mixture for different flavor combinations.
- For a more intense berry flavor, you can add a splash of berry liqueur, such as Chambord or Creme de Cassis, to the mixture before freezing.
- For a smoother sorbet, strain the berry mixture before freezing to remove any seeds or pulp. However, if you prefer a more rustic texture, you can skip this step.
- Store any leftover sorbet in an airtight container in the freezer for up to 1-2 weeks. Allow it to soften slightly at room temperature for a few minutes before serving.

- Berries are packed with antioxidants, including vitamin C and flavonoids, which help protect the body from oxidative stress and inflammation.
- Berry sorbet is naturally low in calories and fat, making it a guilt-free dessert option for those watching their calorie intake.
- Berries have a high water content, which helps keep you hydrated and contributes to overall hydration levels.
- Berries are a good source of essential vitamins and minerals, including vitamin C, vitamin K, and manganese, which are important for overall health and well-being.
- The fiber content in berries helps promote healthy digestion and regular bowel movements.
- The antioxidants and fiber in berries contribute to heart health by reducing the risk of heart disease and improving cholesterol levels.
- Berries are low in calories and high in fiber, making them a satisfying and filling snack that can help with weight management and appetite control.

Health Benefits

9

INTERNATIONAL FLAVORS

Mediterranean Chicken Skewers

- **Preparation Time**: 20 minutes (plus marinating time)
- **Cooking Time**: 10-15 minutes
- **Total Time**: 30-35 minutes (plus marinating time)

Ingredients

- 1.5 lbs (about 700g) boneless, skinless chicken breasts or thighs, cut into bite-sized pieces
- 1/4 cup olive oil
- 3 cloves garlic, minced
- 1 tablespoon lemon juice
- 1 teaspoon lemon zest
- 1 teaspoon dried oregano
- 1 teaspoon dried thyme
- 1 teaspoon dried rosemary
- 1/2 teaspoon paprika
- 1/2 teaspoon ground cumin
- Salt and black pepper, to taste
- Cherry tomatoes, red onion wedges, and bell pepper chunks for skewering

Procedures

1. In a large mixing bowl, whisk together the olive oil, minced garlic, lemon juice, lemon zest, dried oregano, dried thyme, dried rosemary, paprika, ground cumin, salt, and black pepper until well combined.
2. Add the chicken pieces to the bowl with the marinade and toss until evenly coated. Cover the bowl with plastic wrap or transfer the mixture to a resealable plastic bag. Place it in the refrigerator and let the chicken marinate for at least 1-2 hours, or preferably overnight, to allow the flavors to meld and the chicken to tenderize.
3. Preheat an outdoor grill or grill pan over medium-high heat. If using wooden skewers, soak them in water for at least 30 minutes to prevent them from burning.
4. Thread the marinated chicken pieces onto the skewers, alternating with cherry tomatoes, red onion wedges, and bell pepper chunks. Leave a small space between each piece to ensure even cooking.
5. Place the assembled skewers on the preheated grill and cook for 5-7 minutes per side, or until the chicken is cooked through and has grill marks. Use a meat thermometer to ensure the internal temperature of the chicken reaches 165°F (75°C).
6. Once cooked, remove the skewers from the grill and transfer them to a serving platter. Garnish with fresh herbs, if desired, and serve hot.
7. Serve the Mediterranean chicken skewers with your favorite sides, such as rice, quinoa, or a Greek salad, and enjoy the delicious flavors of the Mediterranean!

Nutritional Values (per serving, makes 4 servings)

- Calories: 280
- Total Fat: 12g
- Saturated Fat: 2g
- Cholesterol: 120mg
- Sodium: 350mg
- Total Carbohydrates: 5g
- Dietary Fiber: 1g
- Sugars: 1g
- Protein: 36g

Tips for Making Mediterranean Chicken Skewers

- Use boneless, skinless chicken breasts or thighs for the best results. Trim any excess fat from the chicken before cutting it into bite-sized pieces.
- For maximum flavor, marinate the chicken for at least 1-2 hours, or preferably overnight. This allows the chicken to absorb the flavors of the marinade and become more tender.
- Cut the chicken pieces into uniform sizes to ensure even cooking. This helps prevent smaller pieces from overcooking while waiting for larger pieces to cook through.
- Be careful not to overcook the chicken, as it can become dry and tough. Use a meat thermometer to check for doneness, and remove the skewers from the grill as soon as the internal temperature reaches 165°F (75°C).
- Feel free to customize the skewers by adding other vegetables, such as zucchini, mushrooms, or eggplant, to suit your taste preferences.
- Serve the Mediterranean chicken skewers with a side of tzatziki sauce or hummus for dipping, or drizzle them with a squeeze of lemon juice for extra flavor.

Health Benefits

- Chicken is a rich source of lean protein, which is essential for muscle growth and repair, as well as overall health and well-being.
- Olive oil, a key ingredient in the marinade, is rich in monounsaturated fats, which have been shown to promote heart health and reduce the risk of heart disease.
- Herbs and spices like oregano, thyme, rosemary, and paprika are rich in antioxidants, which help protect the body from oxidative stress and inflammation.
- Bell peppers, onions, and tomatoes are rich in vitamins and minerals, including vitamin C, vitamin A, and potassium, which are important for overall health and immune function.
- Mediterranean chicken skewers are naturally low in carbohydrates, making them suitable for low-carb or ketogenic diets.
- Lean protein and vegetables are filling and satisfying, making Mediterranean chicken skewers a great option for those looking to manage their weight or increase their protein intake.

Asian-Inspired Stir-Fry

Preparation Time: 15 minutes
Cooking Time: 10-15 minutes
Total Time: 25-30 minutes

Ingredients

For the Stir-Fry:
- 1 lb (450g) boneless, skinless chicken breast or tofu, cut into bite-sized pieces
- 2 tablespoons vegetable oil (such as canola or peanut oil)
- 1 red bell pepper, thinly sliced
- 1 yellow bell pepper, thinly sliced
- 1 cup broccoli florets
- 1 cup snap peas
- 1 medium carrot, julienned
- 3 green onions, sliced
- 3 cloves garlic, minced
- 1 tablespoon ginger, minced

For the Sauce:
- 1/4 cup low-sodium soy sauce
- 2 tablespoons hoisin sauce
- 1 tablespoon rice vinegar
- 1 tablespoon honey or maple syrup
- 1 teaspoon sesame oil
- 1 teaspoon cornstarch mixed with 2 tablespoons water (optional, for thickening)

Optional Garnishes:
- Sesame seeds
- Fresh cilantro, chopped
- Sliced green onions

Procedures

1. Cut the chicken breast or tofu into bite-sized pieces. Prepare the vegetables by slicing the bell peppers, julienning the carrot, and cutting the broccoli into florets. Mince the garlic and ginger, and slice the green onions.
2. In a small bowl, whisk together the soy sauce, hoisin sauce, rice vinegar, honey or maple syrup, and sesame oil. If you prefer a thicker sauce, add the cornstarch slurry (cornstarch mixed with water) to the sauce mixture.
3. Heat 1 tablespoon of vegetable oil in a large wok or skillet over medium-high heat. Add the chicken or tofu and cook for 4-5 minutes, stirring occasionally, until the chicken is browned and cooked through or the tofu is golden and crispy. Remove from the wok and set aside.
4. Add the remaining tablespoon of vegetable oil to the wok. Add the minced garlic and ginger, and stir-fry for about 30 seconds until fragrant. Add the bell peppers, broccoli, snap peas, and carrots. Stir-fry for 3-4 minutes until the vegetables are tender-crisp.
5. Return the cooked chicken or tofu to the wok with the vegetables. Pour the sauce over the stir-fry and toss to combine. Cook for an additional 2-3 minutes until everything is heated through and the sauce has thickened slightly.

6. Transfer the stir-fry to serving plates or a large serving dish. Garnish with sesame seeds, chopped cilantro, and sliced green onions if desired.
7. Serve the Asian-inspired stir-fry over steamed rice, quinoa, or noodles, and enjoy a healthy and flavorful meal!

Nutritional Values (per serving, makes 4 servings)

- Calories: 300
- Total Fat: 12g
- Saturated Fat: 2g
- Cholesterol: 60mg (if using chicken)
- Sodium: 800mg
- Total Carbohydrates: 25g
- Dietary Fiber: 5g
- Sugars: 10g
- Protein: 25g

Tips for Making Asian-Inspired Stir-Fry

- Stir-frying is done at high heat, so make sure to preheat your wok or skillet properly. This ensures the ingredients cook quickly and retain their vibrant color and crunch.
- Have all your ingredients prepped and ready to go before you start cooking. Stir-frying happens quickly, and you won't have time to chop or measure once you begin.
- Cut vegetables and proteins into uniform sizes to ensure even cooking. This helps prevent some pieces from being overcooked while others are undercooked.
- Fresh vegetables and herbs add the best flavor and texture to your stir-fry. Avoid using canned or frozen vegetables if possible.
- Feel free to use your favorite vegetables and proteins. Shrimp, beef, or pork can be used instead of chicken or tofu. Vegetables like mushrooms, bok choy, or zucchini can also be great additions.
- Taste the sauce before adding it to the stir-fry and adjust the seasonings to your liking. You can add more soy sauce for saltiness, honey for sweetness, or rice vinegar for acidity.
- Pair your stir-fry with whole grains like brown rice, quinoa, or whole-wheat noodles for added fiber and nutrients.

Health Benefits

- Chicken or tofu provides a good source of protein, essential for muscle repair, growth, and overall body function.
- The variety of vegetables in the stir-fry contributes a range of vitamins, minerals, and antioxidants, promoting overall health and reducing the risk of chronic diseases.
- This stir-fry is relatively low in calories, making it a suitable option for those looking to manage their weight without compromising on flavor or nutrition.
- The use of vegetable oil and sesame oil provides healthy fats that are beneficial for heart health.
- Vegetables like bell peppers, broccoli, and snap peas add dietary

fiber, which aids in digestion, promotes satiety, and helps maintain stable blood sugar levels.
- Ingredients such as bell peppers, broccoli, and ginger are rich in antioxidants, which protect the body from oxidative stress and inflammation.
- Garlic and ginger have immune-boosting properties, helping the body fight off infections and illnesses.

Mexican-Style Tofu Tacos

Preparation Time: 20 minutes
Cooking Time: 20 minutes
Total Time: 40 minutes

Ingredients

For the Tofu Filling:
- 1 block (14 oz) firm or extra-firm tofu, pressed and crumbled
- 2 tablespoons olive oil
- 1 small onion, finely chopped
- 2 cloves garlic, minced
- 1 red bell pepper, diced
- 1 tablespoon chili powder
- 1 teaspoon ground cumin
- 1 teaspoon smoked paprika
- 1/2 teaspoon ground coriander
- 1/4 teaspoon cayenne pepper (optional, for extra heat)
- Salt and black pepper, to taste
- 1 tablespoon soy sauce or tamari
- 1/4 cup vegetable broth or water
- Juice of 1 lime

For the Tacos:
- 8 small corn or flour tortillas
- 1 cup shredded lettuce
- 1 cup diced tomatoes
- 1/2 cup diced red onion
- 1/2 cup chopped fresh cilantro
- 1 avocado, sliced or diced
- 1/2 cup vegan sour cream or regular sour cream
- Lime wedges, for serving

Procedures

1. Press the tofu to remove excess moisture. To do this, wrap the tofu block in a clean kitchen towel and place a heavy object, like a cast-iron skillet, on top. Let it sit for about 15-20 minutes. Once pressed, crumble the tofu into small pieces resembling ground meat.
2. In a large skillet, heat the olive oil over medium heat. Add the chopped onion and cook until translucent, about 3-4 minutes. Add the minced garlic and cook for another minute until fragrant.
3. Add the crumbled tofu to the skillet and cook for about 5 minutes, stirring occasionally, until it starts to brown slightly.
4. Add the diced red bell pepper to the skillet and cook for another 2-3 minutes. Stir in the chili powder, ground cumin, smoked paprika, ground coriander, cayenne pepper (if using), salt, and black pepper. Cook for about 1 minute until the spices are fragrant.
5. Stir in the soy sauce or tamari, vegetable broth or water, and lime juice. Reduce the heat to low and let the mixture simmer for about 5-7 minutes, allowing the flavors to meld and the tofu to absorb the seasonings. Adjust the seasoning if needed.
6. While the tofu mixture is simmering, warm the tortillas in a dry skillet over medium heat for about 30 seconds per side or until they are pliable and slightly toasted. Alternatively, you

can wrap the tortillas in a damp paper towel and microwave them for 30-60 seconds.
7. To assemble the tacos, place a generous spoonful of the tofu filling onto each tortilla. Top with shredded lettuce, diced tomatoes, diced red onion, chopped cilantro, and avocado slices. Drizzle with vegan or regular sour cream and serve with lime wedges on the side.
8. Serve the Mexican-style tofu tacos immediately and enjoy the burst of flavors in every bite!

Nutritional Values (per serving, makes 4 servings)

- Calories: 280
- Total Fat: 16g
- Saturated Fat: 2.5g
- Cholesterol: 0mg
- Sodium: 550mg
- Total Carbohydrates: 24g
- Dietary Fiber: 8g
- Sugars: 4g
- Protein: 12g

Tips for Making Mexican-Style Tofu Tacos

- Properly pressing the tofu removes excess moisture, which helps it absorb more flavor and achieve a better texture. If you're short on time, you can buy pre-pressed tofu or use a tofu press for convenience.
- Feel free to customize the toppings based on your preferences. Other great additions include pickled jalapeños, shredded cheese (vegan or regular), or salsa.
- Tailor the spice level to your taste by adjusting the amount of chili powder and cayenne pepper. For a milder version, omit the cayenne pepper and reduce the chili powder.
- The tofu filling can be made ahead of time and stored in the refrigerator for up to 3 days. Reheat it gently on the stovetop before serving.
- Complement the tacos with sides like Mexican rice, refried beans, or a simple corn salad for a complete meal.
- Use corn tortillas instead of flour tortillas to make the tacos gluten-free. Ensure that all other ingredients, such as soy sauce, are also gluten-free.

Health Benefits

- Tofu is a great plant-based source of protein, providing all the essential amino acids needed for muscle repair and growth.
- Tofu is packed with essential nutrients such as calcium, iron, and magnesium, which are vital for bone health, oxygen transport, and muscle function.
- Tofu contains isoflavones and other compounds that can help reduce cholesterol levels and promote heart health.
- The combination of protein and fiber in these tacos helps promote satiety and can aid in weight management by keeping you full longer.

- The vegetables and spices in the tacos are rich in antioxidants, which help protect the body against oxidative stress and inflammation.
- The fiber from the vegetables and tofu supports healthy digestion and regular bowel movements.
- Tofu fortified with calcium provides a good source of calcium, which is essential for maintaining strong bones and preventing osteoporosis.

Indian Spiced Lentils

Preparation Time: 10 minutes
Cooking Time: 40 minutes
Total Time: 50 minutes

Ingredients

For the Lentils:
- 1 cup split red lentils (masoor dal), rinsed well
- 4 cups water
- 1 teaspoon turmeric powder
- 1 teaspoon salt

For the Spice Tempering:
- 2 tablespoons ghee or vegetable oil
- 1 teaspoon cumin seeds
- 1 medium onion, finely chopped
- 2 cloves garlic, minced
- 1 inch piece ginger, minced
- 1-2 green chilies, slit (optional, for heat)
- 1 large tomato, finely chopped
- 1 teaspoon ground coriander
- 1/2 teaspoon ground cumin
- 1/2 teaspoon garam masala
- 1/2 teaspoon red chili powder (optional, for extra heat)
- 1 teaspoon salt (or to taste)
- Fresh cilantro, chopped, for garnish
- Juice of 1 lemon or lime

Procedures

1. In a large pot, combine the rinsed lentils, water, turmeric powder, and salt. Bring to a boil over medium-high heat. Reduce the heat to medium-low, cover partially, and simmer for about 20-25 minutes, or until the lentils are soft and fully cooked. Stir occasionally to prevent sticking. Once cooked, use a whisk or spoon to mash the lentils slightly for a creamy consistency.
2. In a separate pan, heat the ghee or vegetable oil over medium heat. Add the cumin seeds and cook until they start to sizzle and become aromatic, about 1 minute.
3. Add the finely chopped onion to the pan and sauté until golden brown, about 5-7 minutes. Add the minced garlic, ginger, and green chilies, and cook for another 1-2 minutes until fragrant.
4. Add the chopped tomato to the pan and cook until it softens and the oil starts to separate from the tomato mixture, about 5 minutes. Stir in the ground coriander, ground cumin, garam masala, and red chili powder (if using). Cook for another 2-3 minutes to allow the spices to release their flavors.
5. Pour the spice tempering into the pot with the cooked lentils. Stir well to combine and simmer for another 10 minutes, allowing the flavors to meld together. Adjust the salt to taste.
6. Stir in the lemon or lime juice and garnish with fresh cilantro. Serve hot with steamed basmati rice or Indian bread like naan or roti.

Nutritional Values (per serving, makes 4 servings)

- Calories: 250
- Total Fat: 6g
- Saturated Fat: 2g
- Cholesterol: 0mg
- Sodium: 950mg
- Total Carbohydrates: 35g
- Dietary Fiber: 10g
- Sugars: 5g
- Protein: 12g

Tips for Making Indian Spiced Lentils

- Rinsing lentils well before cooking helps remove dust and reduces foam formation during cooking.
- Customize the heat level by adjusting the amount of green chilies and red chili powder. For a milder dish, omit the chilies or use less.
- For a thicker dal, use less water or cook the lentils a bit longer. For a soupier consistency, add more water as needed.
- Freshly ground spices enhance the flavor of the dish. If possible, grind whole spices just before using them.
- Fresh cilantro and a squeeze of lemon or lime juice add brightness and freshness to the dish.
- Experiment with different types of lentils (such as yellow lentils or green lentils) or add vegetables like spinach, carrots, or tomatoes for added nutrition.

Health Benefits

- Lentils are an excellent plant-based source of protein, making them a great alternative to meat.
- Lentils provide a significant amount of dietary fiber, which promotes healthy digestion and helps regulate blood sugar levels.
- Lentils are packed with essential nutrients, including iron, folate, and magnesium, which support various bodily functions, from energy production to maintaining healthy blood cells.
- This dish is naturally low in fat, especially if you use a minimal amount of oil or ghee.
- The fiber, folate, and potassium in lentils contribute to heart health by reducing cholesterol levels and supporting healthy blood pressure.
- The complex carbohydrates and fiber in lentils help stabilize blood sugar levels, making them beneficial for people with diabetes.
- Spices such as turmeric, cumin, and coriander have antioxidant properties that help combat inflammation and protect against chronic diseases.

10

COMFORT FOOD MAKEOVERS

Cauliflower Mac and Cheese

Preparation Time: 15 minutes
Cooking Time: 30 minutes
Total Time: 45 minutes

Ingredients

For the Cauliflower:
- 1 large head of cauliflower, cut into florets

- 1 tablespoon olive oil
- Salt and black pepper, to taste

For the Cheese Sauce:
- 2 tablespoons unsalted butter
- 2 tablespoons all-purpose flour
- 2 cups milk (whole, 2%, or unsweetened almond milk)
- 1 teaspoon mustard powder
- 1 teaspoon garlic powder
- 1 teaspoon onion powder
- 1/2 teaspoon paprika
- 1/2 teaspoon salt (or to taste)
- 1/4 teaspoon black pepper
- 2 cups shredded sharp cheddar cheese
- 1/2 cup grated Parmesan cheese

Optional Toppings:
- 1/4 cup panko breadcrumbs
- 2 tablespoons melted butter
- 1 tablespoon chopped fresh parsley

Procedures

1. Preheat your oven to 400°F (200°C). Place the cauliflower florets on a baking sheet, drizzle with olive oil, and season with salt and black pepper. Toss to coat evenly.
2. Roast in the preheated oven for 20-25 minutes, or until the cauliflower is tender and lightly browned. Remove from the oven and set aside.
3. In a medium saucepan, melt the butter over medium heat. Once melted, add the flour and whisk continuously for about 2 minutes to form a roux, which will thicken the sauce.
4. Gradually whisk in the milk, making sure to smooth out any lumps. Continue to cook and whisk for about 5-7 minutes, or until the sauce thickens and starts to bubble.
5. Add the mustard powder, garlic powder, onion powder, paprika, salt, and black pepper. Stir to combine and cook for another 1-2 minutes.
6. Reduce the heat to low and gradually stir in the shredded cheddar cheese and Parmesan cheese until fully melted and smooth.
7. Place the roasted cauliflower florets into a large mixing bowl. Pour the cheese sauce over the cauliflower and stir gently to coat the florets evenly.
8. If you prefer a crunchy topping, mix the panko breadcrumbs with the melted butter in a small bowl. Sprinkle the breadcrumb mixture over the cauliflower and cheese.
9. Transfer the cauliflower mac and cheese to a baking dish. If using the breadcrumb topping, spread it evenly over the top.
10. Bake in the preheated oven at 400°F (200°C) for 10-15 minutes, or until the top is golden and crispy.
11. Remove from the oven and let it cool slightly. Garnish with chopped fresh parsley if desired. Serve warm.

Nutritional Values (per serving, makes 6 servings)

- Calories: 270
- Total Fat: 18g
- Saturated Fat: 11g
- Cholesterol: 55mg

- Sodium: 580mg
- Total Carbohydrates: 12g
- Dietary Fiber: 3g
- Sugars: 5g
- Protein: 14g

Tips for Making Cauliflower Mac and Cheese

- Ensure the cauliflower florets are cut to a uniform size for even roasting and cooking.
- For a different flavor profile, try using a mix of cheeses such as Gruyère, mozzarella, or Monterey Jack.
- Incorporate other vegetables like broccoli or spinach for added nutrition and variety.
- Add a dash of hot sauce or a pinch of red pepper flakes to the cheese sauce for a spicy kick.
- Use a gluten-free flour blend for the roux and gluten-free breadcrumbs for the topping to make the dish suitable for those with gluten sensitivities.
- For a lighter version, use low-fat milk and reduce the amount of cheese.

Health Benefits

- Swapping pasta for cauliflower reduces the carbohydrate content, making it suitable for low-carb diets.
- Cauliflower is an excellent source of vitamins C and K, as well as folate, which are essential for overall health.
- The fiber content in cauliflower promotes digestive health and helps maintain a healthy gut.
- Cauliflower contains antioxidants that help reduce inflammation and protect against chronic diseases.
- The cheese provides calcium and phosphorus, which are important for maintaining strong bones and teeth.
- This dish is lower in calories compared to traditional mac and cheese, making it a healthier option for those looking to manage their weight.
- The vitamins and antioxidants in cauliflower support a healthy immune system, helping the body fend off infections.

Turkey Meatloaf

Preparation Time: 20 minutes
Cooking Time: 1 hour
Total Time: 1 hour 20 minutes

Ingredients

For the Meatloaf:
- 2 pounds ground turkey
- 1 small onion, finely chopped
- 2 cloves garlic, minced
- 1 small carrot, grated
- 1 small zucchini, grated
- 1 cup whole wheat breadcrumbs
- 1/2 cup milk (or unsweetened almond milk)
- 1/4 cup ketchup
- 2 tablespoons Worcestershire sauce
- 2 tablespoons tomato paste
- 2 large eggs, lightly beaten
- 1 teaspoon dried thyme
- 1 teaspoon dried basil
- 1 teaspoon dried oregano
- 1 teaspoon salt
- 1/2 teaspoon black pepper

For the Glaze:
- 1/2 cup ketchup
- 2 tablespoons brown sugar
- 1 tablespoon apple cider vinegar
- 1 teaspoon Dijon mustard

Procedures
1. Preheat your oven to 350°F (175°C). Line a baking sheet with parchment paper or lightly grease a loaf pan.
2. Finely chop the onion and mince the garlic. Grate the carrot and zucchini. Squeeze out any excess moisture from the grated zucchini using a clean kitchen towel or paper towel.
3. In a large mixing bowl, combine the ground turkey, chopped onion, minced garlic, grated carrot, grated zucchini, whole wheat breadcrumbs, milk, ketchup, Worcestershire sauce, tomato paste, and beaten eggs. Add the dried thyme, basil, oregano, salt, and black pepper. Mix well until all ingredients are thoroughly combined.
4. Transfer the meat mixture to the prepared baking sheet or loaf pan. Shape it into a loaf form if using a baking sheet.
5. In a small bowl, mix together the ketchup, brown sugar, apple cider vinegar, and Dijon mustard. Stir until smooth.
6. Spread half of the glaze evenly over the top of the meatloaf.
7. Bake in the preheated oven for 1 hour. About 10 minutes before the meatloaf is done, remove it from the oven and spread the remaining glaze over the top. Return to the oven and continue baking until the meatloaf is cooked through and the internal temperature reaches 165°F (74°C).
8. Once cooked, remove the meatloaf from the oven and let it rest for 10 minutes before slicing. This allows the juices to redistribute, ensuring a moist meatloaf. Serve warm.

Nutritional Values (per serving, makes 8 servings)

- Calories: 290

- Total Fat: 12g
- Saturated Fat: 3g
- Cholesterol: 125mg
- Sodium: 720mg
- Total Carbohydrates: 20g
- Dietary Fiber: 2g
- Sugars: 7g
- Protein: 25g

Tips for Making Turkey Meatloaf

- Adding grated vegetables like carrot and zucchini helps keep the meatloaf moist. You can also add a bit of finely chopped mushrooms for additional moisture and flavor.
- Mix the ingredients until just combined to avoid a dense meatloaf. Overmixing can result in a tougher texture.
- Allow the meatloaf to rest for about 10 minutes after baking. This helps retain its shape and ensures it stays juicy.
- For a different flavor profile, you can experiment with different types of mustard, such as honey mustard or spicy brown mustard, in the glaze.
- To ensure the meatloaf is fully cooked, use a meat thermometer to check that the internal temperature reaches 165°F (74°C).
- Prepare the meatloaf mixture ahead of time and store it in the refrigerator for up to 24 hours before baking. This can save time on busy days.
- Turkey meatloaf makes excellent leftovers. Store in an airtight container in the refrigerator for up to 3 days, or freeze individual slices for later use.

Health Benefits

- Ground turkey is a lean source of protein, which is essential for muscle building and repair.
- Compared to traditional meatloaf made with beef, turkey meatloaf is lower in saturated fat, which can benefit heart health.
- The addition of vegetables like carrot and zucchini boosts the vitamin and mineral content, providing nutrients such as vitamin A, vitamin C, and potassium.
- Whole wheat breadcrumbs add fiber to the meatloaf, promoting digestive health and helping to maintain healthy blood sugar levels.
- The high protein content helps keep you feeling full longer, which can aid in weight management.
- Garlic and onions contain compounds that support the immune system and have anti-inflammatory properties.
- Turkey is a good source of iron, which is important for producing red blood cells and preventing anemia.

Low-Sodium Beef Stroganoff

Preparation Time: 15 minutes
Cooking Time: 30 minutes
Total Time: 45 minutes

Ingredients

For the Stroganoff:
- 1 pound beef sirloin or tenderloin, cut into thin strips
- 1 tablespoon olive oil
- 1 medium onion, finely chopped
- 2 cloves garlic, minced
- 8 ounces mushrooms, sliced
- 1 cup low-sodium beef broth
- 1 tablespoon Worcestershire sauce (low-sodium if available)
- 1 tablespoon tomato paste (no added salt)
- 1 teaspoon paprika
- 1 teaspoon dried thyme
- 1/2 teaspoon black pepper
- 1/2 cup plain Greek yogurt (or low-fat sour cream)
- 1 tablespoon cornstarch mixed with 2 tablespoons water (optional, for thickening)

For Serving:
- 8 ounces whole wheat egg noodles or brown rice
- Fresh parsley, chopped (for garnish)

Procedures

1. Cut the beef into thin strips and set aside. Finely chop the onion and mince the garlic. Slice the mushrooms.
2. Heat the olive oil in a large skillet over medium-high heat. Add the beef strips and cook until browned on all sides, about 3-4 minutes. Remove the beef from the skillet and set aside.
3. In the same skillet, add the chopped onion and garlic. Sauté until the onion becomes translucent, about 3 minutes. Add the sliced mushrooms and cook until they release their moisture and become tender, about 5 minutes.
4. Add the low-sodium beef broth, Worcestershire sauce, tomato paste, paprika, dried thyme, and black pepper to the skillet. Stir to combine and bring to a simmer. Let the sauce cook for about 5 minutes to allow the flavors to meld together.
5. If you prefer a thicker sauce, stir the cornstarch mixture into the skillet. Cook, stirring constantly, until the sauce has thickened to your desired consistency.
6. Return the cooked beef to the skillet and stir to coat with the sauce. Reduce the heat to low and let it simmer for about 5 minutes to heat the beef through.
7. Remove the skillet from the heat and stir in the plain Greek yogurt. Mix until well combined and the sauce is creamy.
8. While the Stroganoff is simmering, cook the whole wheat egg noodles or

brown rice according to package instructions. Drain and set aside.
9. Serve the Beef Stroganoff over the cooked noodles or rice. Garnish with chopped fresh parsley.

Nutritional Values (per serving, makes 4 servings)

- Calories: 350
- Total Fat: 15g
- Saturated Fat: 5g
- Cholesterol: 90mg
- Sodium: 200mg
- Total Carbohydrates: 30g
- Dietary Fiber: 4g
- Sugars: 6g
- Protein: 25g

Tips for Making Low-Sodium Beef Stroganoff

- Use lean cuts of beef like sirloin or tenderloin to reduce the fat content and make the dish healthier.
- Opt for low-sodium beef broth and check the labels on Worcestershire sauce and tomato paste to find low-sodium versions. You can also make homemade beef broth to control the sodium content.
- Use herbs and spices like paprika, thyme, and black pepper to add flavor without relying on salt. Fresh garlic and onions also enhance the taste.
- If you prefer a thicker sauce, use a cornstarch slurry (cornstarch mixed with water) to achieve the desired consistency without adding more fat or calories.
- Plain Greek yogurt can be used instead of sour cream for a healthier, protein-rich alternative that adds creaminess to the sauce.
- Include additional vegetables like bell peppers or spinach for added nutrients and variety.
- Serve the Stroganoff over whole wheat noodles or brown rice to increase fiber content and provide a more balanced meal.

Health Benefits

- This version of Beef Stroganoff is lower in sodium, making it suitable for individuals managing high blood pressure or heart disease.
- Lean beef provides a high-quality source of protein, essential for muscle repair and growth.
- The addition of mushrooms and other vegetables boosts the content of vitamins B and D, as well as minerals like potassium and selenium.
- Using lean cuts of beef and Greek yogurt instead of sour cream reduces the saturated fat content, benefiting heart health.
- Whole wheat noodles or brown rice add dietary fiber, promoting healthy digestion and aiding in maintaining stable blood sugar levels.
- Ingredients like garlic and onions have immune-boosting properties due to their antimicrobial and anti-inflammatory compounds.
- The beef provides essential nutrients like phosphorus and zinc, which are

important for maintaining strong bones and overall health.

Chicken Pot Pie with a Twist

Preparation Time: 30 minutes
Cooking Time: 1 hour
Total Time: 1 hour 30 minutes

Ingredients

For the Filling:
- 2 tablespoons olive oil
- 1 pound boneless, skinless chicken breast, diced
- 1 medium onion, chopped
- 2 cloves garlic, minced
- 2 medium carrots, diced
- 2 celery stalks, diced
- 1 medium sweet potato, peeled and diced
- 1 cup green beans, cut into 1-inch pieces
- 1 cup peas (fresh or frozen)
- 2 cups low-sodium chicken broth
- 1 cup low-fat milk (or unsweetened almond milk)
- 1/4 cup whole wheat flour
- 1 teaspoon dried thyme
- 1 teaspoon dried rosemary
- 1 teaspoon paprika
- 1/2 teaspoon black pepper
- 1/4 teaspoon salt (optional)

For the Crust:
- 1 1/2 cups whole wheat flour
- 1/2 cup rolled oats
- 1 teaspoon baking powder
- 1/2 teaspoon salt
- 1/2 cup cold unsalted butter, cubed
- 1/2 cup low-fat Greek yogurt
- 1/4 cup cold water

Procedures

1. Heat the olive oil in a large skillet over medium-high heat. Add the diced chicken and cook until browned and cooked through, about 5-7 minutes. Remove the chicken from the skillet and set aside.
2. In the same skillet, add the chopped onion and minced garlic. Sauté until the onion becomes translucent, about 3 minutes.
3. Add the diced carrots, celery, and sweet potato. Cook for about 5 minutes until they start to soften.
4. Stir in the green beans and peas, cooking for another 2-3 minutes.
5. Sprinkle the whole wheat flour over the vegetables in the skillet. Stir well to coat the vegetables and cook for about 1-2 minutes to remove the raw flour taste.
6. Gradually pour in the low-sodium chicken broth and low-fat milk, stirring constantly to avoid lumps.
7. Add the dried thyme, dried rosemary, paprika, black pepper, and salt (if using). Bring the mixture to a simmer and cook until it thickens, about 5 minutes.
8. Return the cooked chicken to the skillet and stir to combine. Remove from heat and set aside.
9. In a large bowl, combine the whole wheat flour, rolled oats, baking powder, and salt.

10. Add the cold, cubed butter and use a pastry cutter or your fingers to work it into the flour mixture until it resembles coarse crumbs.
11. Stir in the Greek yogurt, then add the cold water a little at a time, mixing until the dough comes together.
12. Form the dough into a ball, cover with plastic wrap, and refrigerate for at least 30 minutes.
13. Preheat your oven to 375°F (190°C).
14. Roll out the dough on a floured surface to fit the top of your baking dish (or divide for individual servings).
15. Pour the chicken and vegetable filling into a baking dish. Place the rolled-out dough over the filling, trimming any excess and crimping the edges to seal.
16. Cut a few small slits in the top of the crust to allow steam to escape.
17. Place the pot pie on a baking sheet to catch any drips. Bake in the preheated oven for 30-35 minutes, or until the crust is golden brown and the filling is bubbling.
18. Let the pot pie cool for about 10 minutes before serving. This allows the filling to set and makes it easier to cut and serve.

Nutritional Values (per serving, makes 6 servings)

- Calories: 420
- Total Fat: 16g
- Saturated Fat: 6g
- Cholesterol: 70mg
- Sodium: 350mg
- Total Carbohydrates: 45g
- Dietary Fiber: 8g
- Sugars: 8g
- Protein: 26g

Tips for Making Chicken Pot Pie with a Twist

- Fresh vegetables and herbs provide the best flavor and nutritional benefits. However, you can also use frozen vegetables if fresh ones are not available.
- The filling can be prepared a day in advance and stored in the refrigerator. Assemble and bake the pot pie just before serving for the best results.
- Using whole wheat flour and rolled oats in the crust increases the fiber content and adds a pleasant, nutty flavor.
- You can substitute the sweet potato with regular potato or butternut squash, and the green beans with broccoli or asparagus.
- Choose low-sodium broth and avoid adding extra salt to control the sodium content.
- Feel free to add more vegetables like bell peppers, spinach, or kale for added nutrients and variety.
- For a lighter version, you can use phyllo dough or a single top crust instead of a traditional double crust.

Health Benefits

- The chicken provides a lean source of protein, essential for muscle repair and growth.

- Whole wheat flour, oats, and a variety of vegetables contribute to the high fiber content, which aids in digestion and helps maintain stable blood sugar levels.
- Using olive oil and Greek yogurt reduces the saturated fat content, which is beneficial for heart health.
- The vegetables in this recipe provide a range of vitamins and minerals, including vitamins A and C, potassium, and magnesium.
- Ingredients like sweet potatoes and carrots are rich in antioxidants, which help protect the body from damage caused by free radicals.
- The high protein and fiber content help keep you feeling full longer, which can aid in weight management.
- The inclusion of low-fat milk and Greek yogurt adds calcium and vitamin D, important for maintaining strong bones.
- Garlic and onions contain compounds that support the immune system and have anti-inflammatory properties.

11

SPECIAL OCCASION MEALS

Rosemary Lamb Chops

Preparation Time: 15 minutes (plus 30 minutes marinating time)
Cooking Time: 15 minutes

Total Time: 1 hour

Ingredients

For the Lamb Chops:
- 8 lamb chops (approximately 1 inch thick)
- 2 tablespoons fresh rosemary, finely chopped
- 3 cloves garlic, minced
- 1 tablespoon lemon zest
- 2 tablespoons olive oil
- 1 tablespoon fresh lemon juice
- 1 teaspoon black pepper
- 1/2 teaspoon salt (optional)
- Fresh rosemary sprigs (for garnish, optional)
- Lemon wedges (for serving, optional)

Procedures

1. In a small bowl, combine the chopped rosemary, minced garlic, lemon zest, olive oil, lemon juice, black pepper, and salt (if using). Mix well to form a marinade.
2. Place the lamb chops in a shallow dish or a resealable plastic bag. Pour the marinade over the lamb chops, ensuring they are well coated. Cover the dish or seal the bag and refrigerate for at least 30 minutes, or up to 2 hours for more intense flavor.
3. If using a grill, preheat it to medium-high heat. If using a skillet, preheat it over medium-high heat until hot.
4. Remove the lamb chops from the marinade, allowing any excess to drip off. Place the chops on the grill or in the hot skillet.
5. Cook the lamb chops for about 3-4 minutes per side for medium-rare, or longer depending on your preferred level of doneness. Use a meat thermometer to check the internal temperature (145°F for medium-rare, 160°F for medium).
6. Transfer the cooked lamb chops to a plate and cover with foil. Let them rest for about 5 minutes to allow the juices to redistribute.
7. Garnish the lamb chops with fresh rosemary sprigs and serve with lemon wedges. Pair with your favorite sides, such as roasted vegetables or a fresh salad.

Nutritional Values (per serving, makes 4 servings)

- Calories: 450
- Total Fat: 30g
- Saturated Fat: 12g
- Cholesterol: 115mg
- Sodium: 300mg
- Total Carbohydrates: 2g
- Dietary Fiber: 1g
- Sugars: 0g
- Protein: 35g

Tips for Making Rosemary Lamb Chops

- For the best flavor and texture, choose lamb chops that are fresh and of high quality. Grass-fed lamb is a good option for its enhanced flavor and nutritional profile.
- Allow the lamb chops to marinate for at least 30 minutes to let the flavors

- penetrate the meat. If you have more time, marinate for up to 2 hours.
- Use a meat thermometer to check for doneness. Lamb is best enjoyed medium-rare to medium, as overcooking can make it tough and dry.
- Let the lamb chops rest after cooking to retain their juices and enhance the tenderness of the meat.
- If using a grill, ensure it is properly preheated to achieve a nice sear on the lamb chops. You can also add a bit of wood chips to the grill for a smoky flavor.
- If using a skillet, ensure it is hot before adding the lamb chops. A cast-iron skillet works well for achieving a good sear.
- Serve the lamb chops with sides that complement the rich flavor of the meat, such as garlic mashed potatoes, roasted Brussels sprouts, or a quinoa salad.

Health Benefits

- Lamb is a great source of high-quality protein, which is essential for muscle repair, growth, and overall body function.
- Lamb provides important nutrients like vitamin B12, iron, zinc, and selenium, which are vital for energy production, immune function, and cognitive health.
- While lamb does contain saturated fat, it also provides healthy monounsaturated fats and omega-3 fatty acids, particularly if it's grass-fed. These fats can help maintain healthy cholesterol levels and support cardiovascular health.
- Rosemary is rich in antioxidants and anti-inflammatory compounds that can help protect the body from oxidative stress and inflammation.
- Garlic and lemon, included in the marinade, are known to aid digestion and provide antimicrobial benefits.
- The high levels of zinc and phosphorus in lamb are essential for maintaining strong bones and teeth.
- The zinc content in lamb plays a crucial role in supporting the immune system, helping to ward off infections and illnesses.

Stuffed Chicken Breast with Spinach and Cheese

Preparation Time: 20 minutes
Cooking Time: 25 minutes
Total Time: 45 minutes

Ingredients

For the Chicken:
- 4 boneless, skinless chicken breasts
- 1 tablespoon olive oil
- 1 teaspoon paprika
- 1 teaspoon garlic powder
- 1 teaspoon onion powder
- 1/2 teaspoon black pepper
- 1/2 teaspoon salt (optional)

For the Filling:
- 2 cups fresh spinach, chopped
- 1/2 cup ricotta cheese
- 1/2 cup shredded mozzarella cheese
- 1/4 cup grated Parmesan cheese
- 2 cloves garlic, minced
- 1 tablespoon fresh basil, chopped (or 1 teaspoon dried basil)
- 1 tablespoon fresh parsley, chopped (or 1 teaspoon dried parsley)
- 1/4 teaspoon black pepper
- 1/4 teaspoon salt (optional)

Procedures

1. Preheat your oven to 375°F (190°C).
2. Place the chicken breasts on a cutting board. Using a sharp knife, cut a pocket into each chicken breast by slicing horizontally, being careful not to cut all the way through.
3. In a medium bowl, combine the chopped spinach, ricotta cheese, shredded mozzarella cheese, grated Parmesan cheese, minced garlic, chopped basil, chopped parsley, black pepper, and salt (if using). Mix well until all ingredients are thoroughly combined.
4. Spoon the spinach and cheese mixture into the pocket of each chicken breast, distributing the filling evenly among the four breasts. Secure the opening with toothpicks to keep the filling inside during cooking.
5. In a small bowl, mix together the paprika, garlic powder, onion powder, black pepper, and salt (if using). Rub the olive oil over the stuffed chicken breasts, then sprinkle the seasoning mixture evenly over all sides of the chicken.
6. Heat an ovenproof skillet over medium-high heat. Add the stuffed chicken breasts and sear for 2-3 minutes on each side, until golden brown.
7. Transfer the skillet to the preheated oven and bake for 20-25 minutes, or until the chicken is cooked through and the internal temperature reaches 165°F (74°C).
8. Remove the chicken from the oven and let it rest for 5 minutes before serving. Remove the toothpicks and

slice each breast into medallions for a beautiful presentation. Serve with your favorite sides, such as roasted vegetables or a fresh salad.

Nutritional Values (per serving, makes 4 servings)

- Calories: 350
- Total Fat: 18g
- Saturated Fat: 8g
- Cholesterol: 110mg
- Sodium: 500mg
- Total Carbohydrates: 4g
- Dietary Fiber: 1g
- Sugars: 1g
- Protein: 41g

Tips for Making Stuffed Chicken Breast with Spinach and Cheese

- Use large, evenly-sized chicken breasts for easy stuffing and even cooking.
- Use toothpicks to secure the chicken breasts after stuffing to prevent the filling from spilling out during cooking. Remember to remove them before serving.
- Searing the chicken breasts before baking adds a nice golden crust and enhances the flavor. An ovenproof skillet is ideal for this step.
- Experiment with different cheeses like feta or goat cheese for a different flavor profile. You can also add other vegetables like sun-dried tomatoes or mushrooms to the filling.
- Use a meat thermometer to ensure the chicken is cooked through. The internal temperature should reach 165°F (74°C).
- Allow the chicken to rest for a few minutes after baking to retain its juices, resulting in a moister and more flavorful dish.

Health Benefits

- Chicken breast is an excellent source of lean protein, essential for muscle repair, growth, and overall body function.
- Spinach is packed with vitamins A, C, and K, as well as iron, calcium, and magnesium, which are important for bone health, immune function, and energy production.
- Olive oil, used in this recipe, is rich in monounsaturated fats, which are beneficial for heart health and can help reduce bad cholesterol levels.
- This dish is low in carbohydrates, making it suitable for low-carb or keto diets.
- The cheeses used in the filling provide calcium and phosphorus, essential for maintaining strong bones and teeth.
- Spinach and herbs like basil and parsley contain antioxidants that help protect the body from oxidative stress and inflammation.
- The high protein content and low-calorie nature of this dish can help keep you full and satisfied, supporting weight management efforts.
- Garlic, used in the filling, has been shown to promote digestive health

and has natural antimicrobial properties.

Seared Scallops with Lemon Butter

Preparation Time: 10 minutes
Cooking Time: 10 minutes
Total Time: 20 minutes

Ingredients

For the Scallops:
- 1 pound sea scallops (about 12-16 scallops)
- 2 tablespoons olive oil
- 1/2 teaspoon salt
- 1/2 teaspoon black pepper

For the Lemon Butter Sauce:
- 3 tablespoons unsalted butter
- 1 clove garlic, minced
- 1 tablespoon fresh lemon juice
- 1 teaspoon lemon zest
- 1 tablespoon fresh parsley, chopped
- 1/4 teaspoon salt
- 1/4 teaspoon black pepper

Procedures

1. Rinse the scallops under cold water and pat them dry with paper towels. Remove the small side muscle from each scallop if it's still attached.
2. Season the scallops on both sides with salt and black pepper.
3. Heat a large skillet over medium-high heat. Add the olive oil and let it get hot until it starts to shimmer but not smoke.
4. Place the scallops in the skillet in a single layer, making sure they are not touching each other. Cook without moving them for about 2-3 minutes, until the bottom is golden brown.
5. Carefully flip the scallops and cook for another 2-3 minutes, or until the second side is golden brown and the scallops are opaque in the center.
6. Remove the scallops from the skillet and set them aside on a plate.
7. In the same skillet, lower the heat to medium and add the butter. Once the butter has melted, add the minced garlic and sauté for about 30 seconds until fragrant.
8. Add the lemon juice, lemon zest, salt, and black pepper. Stir to combine and let the sauce simmer for 1 minute.
9. Return the scallops to the skillet and spoon the lemon butter sauce over them. Cook for an additional 1-2 minutes to heat the scallops through and coat them in the sauce.
10. Garnish with fresh parsley and serve immediately. Pair with a side of sautéed vegetables or a light salad for a complete meal.

Nutritional Values (per serving, makes 4 servings)

- Calories: 220
- Total Fat: 15g
- Saturated Fat: 6g
- Cholesterol: 50mg
- Sodium: 620mg
- Total Carbohydrates: 3g
- Dietary Fiber: 0g
- Sugars: 0g

- Protein: 18g

Tips for Making Seared Scallops with Lemon Butter

- Fresh, dry-packed scallops are best for this recipe. Avoid wet-packed scallops that are treated with chemicals, as they won't sear as well.
- Make sure the scallops are thoroughly dried before searing. Excess moisture will prevent a good sear and can cause splattering in the pan.
- Ensure the skillet is hot before adding the scallops. This helps achieve a nice golden-brown crust.
- Cook the scallops in batches if necessary to avoid overcrowding the pan, which can cause steaming instead of searing.
- Scallops cook quickly. Keep an eye on them and avoid overcooking, which can make them tough and chewy.
- After searing the scallops, deglaze the pan with a splash of white wine or chicken broth before making the lemon butter sauce for added depth of flavor.
- Serve the scallops with sides that complement their delicate flavor, such as asparagus, risotto, or a fresh green salad.

Health Benefits

- Scallops are an excellent source of lean protein, essential for muscle repair and growth.
- Scallops are naturally low in fat, making them a healthy choice for those looking to reduce their fat intake.
- Scallops provide important nutrients such as vitamin B12, iodine, magnesium, and potassium, which support various bodily functions including nerve health, thyroid function, and heart health.
- The omega-3 fatty acids found in scallops can help reduce inflammation and improve cardiovascular health.
- Garlic and lemon used in the sauce have antioxidant properties that help combat oxidative stress and support overall health.
- Low in calories and high in protein, scallops can help keep you full and satisfied, aiding in weight management.
- The calcium and phosphorus in scallops contribute to maintaining strong bones and teeth.
- The nutrients in scallops, including zinc and selenium, play a crucial role in supporting a healthy immune system.

MEAL PLAN

Day 1

Breakfast: Cinnamon Quinoa Porridge
Lunch: Berry Spinach Salad with Lemon Vinaigrette
Dinner: Herb-Crusted Baked Cod
Snack: Baked Kale Chips

Day 2

Breakfast: Green Detox Smoothie
Lunch: Zesty Quinoa and Veggie Salad
Dinner: Grilled Lemon Chicken
Snack: Spicy Roasted Carrots

Day 3

Breakfast: Low-Phosphorus Pancakes
Lunch: Cucumber Dill Salad
Dinner: Garlic and Herb Pork Tenderloin
Snack: Apple Slices with Almond Butter

Day 4

Breakfast: Herb-Infused Egg White Omelet
Lunch: Hearty Vegetable Soup
Dinner: Vegetarian Stuffed Peppers
Snack: Vanilla Chia Seed Pudding

Day 5

Breakfast: Berry Banana Smoothie
Lunch: Chicken and Rice Soup
Dinner: Seared Scallops with Lemon Butter
Snack: Spicy Chickpea Snack

Day 6

Breakfast: Cinnamon Quinoa Porridge
Lunch: Lentil and Sweet Potato Stew
Dinner: Mediterranean Chicken Skewers
Snack: Baked Apple with Cinnamon

Day 7

Breakfast: Berry Spinach Salad with Lemon Vinaigrette
Dinner: Asian-Inspired Stir-Fry
Snack: Garlic Mashed Cauliflower

Day 8

Breakfast: Low-Phosphorus Pancakes
Lunch: Zesty Quinoa and Veggie Salad
Dinner: Mexican-Style Tofu Tacos
Snack: Rice Pudding with Nutmeg

Day 9

Breakfast: Herb-Infused Egg White Omelet
Lunch: Hearty Vegetable Soup
Dinner: Indian Spiced Lentils
Snack: Spicy Roasted Carrots

Day 10

Breakfast: Berry Banana Smoothie
Lunch: Chicken and Rice Soup
Dinner: Cauliflower Mac and Cheese

Snack: Berry Sorbet

Day 11

Breakfast: Cinnamon Quinoa Porridge
Lunch: Lentil and Sweet Potato Stew
Dinner: Turkey Meatloaf
Snack: Apple Slices with Almond Butter

Day 12

Breakfast: Green Detox Smoothie
Lunch: Cucumber Dill Salad
Dinner: Low-Sodium Beef Stroganoff
Snack: Baked Kale Chips

Day 13

Breakfast: Low-Phosphorus Pancakes
Lunch: Berry Spinach Salad with Lemon Vinaigrette
Dinner: Chicken Pot Pie with a Twist
Snack: Vanilla Chia Seed Pudding

Day 14

Breakfast: Herb-Infused Egg White Omelet
Lunch: Zesty Quinoa and Veggie Salad
Dinner: Rosemary Lamb Chops
Snack: Spicy Chickpea Snack

CONCLUSION

Tips for Long-Term Success in Maintaining a Healthier Lifestyle

Adopting a healthier lifestyle is a significant achievement, but maintaining these positive changes in the long term can be challenging. Success requires persistence, flexibility, and a proactive approach to sustaining your well-being. Here are extensive tips to help you achieve long-term success in your journey toward a healthier lifestyle.

1. Set Realistic and Achievable Goals

Start Small: Begin with manageable goals that you can gradually build upon. For example, if you're new to exercise, start with short daily walks and progressively increase the duration and intensity.

SMART Goals: Use the SMART criteria to set goals – Specific, Measurable, Achievable, Relevant, and Time-bound. This framework helps clarify your objectives and track progress effectively.

Celebrate Milestones: Recognize and celebrate small achievements along the way. Celebrating milestones keeps you motivated and provides a sense of accomplishment.

2. Develop a Routine

Consistency is Key: Establish a daily routine that incorporates healthy habits. Consistency helps transform new behaviors into automatic actions.

Plan Ahead: Schedule your workouts, meal prep sessions, and relaxation time. Planning reduces the likelihood of making unhealthy choices during busy or stressful periods.

Adjust as Needed: Life is dynamic, and routines may need adjustments. Be flexible and willing to modify your schedule to accommodate changes while maintaining your commitment to a healthier lifestyle.

3. Prioritize Nutrition

Balanced Diet: Aim for a balanced diet rich in fruits, vegetables, whole grains, lean proteins, and healthy fats. Variety ensures you get a wide range of nutrients.

Portion Control: Be mindful of portion sizes to avoid overeating. Using smaller plates and bowls can help control portions visually.

Mindful Eating: Practice mindful eating by paying attention to hunger and fullness cues. Avoid distractions like TV or smartphones during meals to focus on the experience of eating.

Healthy Snacking: Choose nutritious snacks such as fruits, nuts, or yogurt instead of processed and high-sugar options. Planning snacks can prevent unhealthy impulse eating.

4. Stay Physically Active

Find Enjoyable Activities: Engage in physical activities you enjoy, whether it's dancing, hiking, swimming, or playing a sport. Enjoyable activities are more likely to become long-term habits.

Incorporate Variety: Mix different types of exercise, including cardio, strength training, flexibility, and balance exercises. Variety prevents boredom and works different muscle groups.

Set a Schedule: Dedicate specific times for exercise in your daily routine. Consistency is crucial for maintaining an active lifestyle.

Use Technology: Fitness apps and wearable devices can track your activity levels, set goals, and provide motivation through reminders and progress reports.

5. Focus on Mental and Emotional Health

Stress Management: Incorporate stress-relief practices such as meditation, deep breathing exercises, yoga, or hobbies that you find relaxing.

Social Connections: Maintain strong relationships with family and friends. Social support provides emotional benefits and can help you stay accountable to your health goals.

Positive Mindset: Cultivate a positive attitude by practicing gratitude and focusing on positive aspects of your life. Positive thinking can enhance mental resilience and overall well-being.

Seek Help When Needed: Don't hesitate to seek professional help if you're struggling with mental health issues. Therapists and counselors can provide valuable support and strategies.

6. Get Quality Sleep

Establish a Routine: Create a consistent sleep schedule by going to bed and waking up at the same time every day, even on weekends.

Create a Sleep-Friendly Environment: Ensure your bedroom is dark, quiet, and cool. Invest in a comfortable mattress and pillows.

Limit Screen Time: Avoid screens (phones, tablets, TVs) at least an hour before bedtime. The blue light from screens can interfere with your sleep cycle.

Relaxation Techniques: Develop a pre-sleep routine that includes relaxation techniques such as reading, taking a warm bath, or practicing mindfulness.

7. Stay Hydrated

Drink Water Regularly: Aim to drink at least eight cups of water a day, adjusting for factors like activity level and climate.

Healthy Beverages: Choose water, herbal teas, and other low-calorie beverages. Limit sugary drinks and excessive caffeine.

Hydration Reminders: Set reminders to drink water throughout the day, especially if you're busy or tend to forget.

Flavor Enhancements: Add natural flavors to your water, such as slices of fruit or herbs, to make it more appealing.

8. Avoid Harmful Habits

Limit Alcohol: Consume alcohol in moderation. For women, this means up to one drink per day, and for men, up to two drinks per day.

Quit Smoking: Seek resources and support to quit smoking. This could include nicotine replacement therapy, counseling, or support groups.

Avoid Recreational Drugs: Refrain from using recreational drugs, and seek help if you struggle with substance abuse.

Healthy Substitutions: Replace harmful habits with positive activities that promote well-being, such as exercise, hobbies, or spending time with loved ones.

9. Monitor Your Progress

Track Your Goals: Keep a journal or use an app to track your progress towards your health goals. Recording your activities, meals, and feelings can provide insights and help you stay accountable.

Self-Reflection: Regularly reflect on your progress and identify areas for improvement. Adjust your goals and strategies as needed.

Celebrate Successes: Acknowledge and celebrate your achievements, no matter how small. Positive reinforcement can boost motivation and confidence.

10. Stay Informed and Educated

Ongoing Learning: Continuously educate yourself about health and wellness through reputable sources such as books, articles, and professional advice.

Stay Updated: Keep up with the latest health guidelines and recommendations from credible organizations like the CDC, WHO, or your healthcare provider.

Seek Professional Guidance: Consult with healthcare professionals, nutritionists, or fitness trainers for personalized advice and support.

11. Build a Support System

Find a Buddy: Partner with a friend or family member who shares similar health goals. Mutual support can enhance accountability and motivation.

Join a Community: Engage in community groups or online forums focused on health and wellness. Sharing experiences and tips can provide valuable support.

Family Involvement: Involve your family in your health journey. Making lifestyle changes together can foster a supportive environment and improve everyone's well-being.

12. Practice Patience and Persistence

Be Patient: Understand that significant changes take time. Patience is crucial as you work towards long-term health goals.

Stay Persistent: Persistence is key to overcoming setbacks. Keep pushing forward even when progress seems slow or challenges arise.

Learn from Setbacks: View setbacks as learning opportunities rather than failures. Analyze what went wrong and adjust your strategies accordingly.

Staying Motivated and Inspired

Maintaining motivation and inspiration is crucial for achieving long-term success in adopting and sustaining a healthier lifestyle. Whether you're aiming to improve your diet, increase physical activity, or enhance overall well-being, staying motivated can be challenging, especially when faced with obstacles and setbacks. Here, we will explore various strategies and techniques to help you stay motivated and inspired on your health journey.

1. Set Clear and Meaningful Goals

Identify Your 'Why': Understand the deeper reasons behind your health goals. Whether it's improving your quality of life, setting a good example for your children, or managing a health condition, having a clear and personal motivation can fuel your commitment.

Break Down Goals: Divide larger goals into smaller, manageable steps. Achieving these smaller milestones provides a sense of accomplishment and keeps you motivated.

Visualize Success: Regularly visualize your success and the benefits that come with achieving your goals. This mental imagery can reinforce your commitment and boost motivation.

Use the SMART Framework: Ensure your goals are Specific, Measurable, Achievable, Relevant, and Time-bound. This clarity helps in maintaining focus and tracking progress.

2. Create a Supportive Environment

Surround Yourself with Positivity: Spend time with people who support and encourage your health goals. Positive influences can keep you motivated and provide a support network.

Eliminate Temptations: Remove unhealthy foods and habits from your environment. A supportive environment minimizes temptations and promotes healthier choices.

Join Groups or Classes: Participate in fitness classes, cooking groups, or online forums focused on health and wellness. Shared experiences and camaraderie can enhance motivation.

Involve Family and Friends: Engage your family and friends in your health journey. Their involvement can provide additional support and accountability.

3. Track Your Progress

Keep a Journal: Record your activities, meals, emotions, and progress. Journaling helps you reflect on your journey, identify patterns, and celebrate successes.

Use Technology: Utilize fitness trackers, apps, and online tools to monitor your progress. These tools provide data and feedback that can boost motivation.

Set Regular Check-ins: Schedule regular check-ins to assess your progress. Reflect on what's working and what needs adjustment.

Celebrate Achievements: Recognize and celebrate your milestones, no matter how small. Celebrations reinforce positive behavior and motivate you to keep going.

4. Stay Educated and Inspired

Read and Research: Stay informed about health and wellness by reading books, articles, and blogs. Knowledge empowers you to make better decisions and stay motivated.

Follow Inspirational Figures: Follow health and fitness influencers, motivational speakers, or experts who inspire you. Their content can provide daily motivation and new ideas.

Attend Workshops and Seminars: Participate in health and wellness workshops or seminars. Learning new techniques and information can reinvigorate your commitment.

Explore New Interests: Try new activities, recipes, or fitness routines. Variety keeps your routine exciting and prevents boredom.

5. Develop Resilience and Adaptability

Embrace Setbacks: Accept that setbacks are a natural part of any journey. Instead of getting discouraged, view them as learning opportunities.

Adapt Your Plan: Be flexible and willing to adjust your goals and strategies as needed. Adaptability ensures you stay on track despite challenges.

Focus on Progress, Not Perfection: Strive for progress rather than perfection. Every positive change, no matter how small, contributes to your overall goal.

Practice Self-Compassion: Be kind to yourself. Treat yourself with the same compassion and understanding you would offer a friend.

6. Incorporate Fun and Enjoyment

Choose Enjoyable Activities: Engage in physical activities and hobbies you enjoy. Enjoyment increases the likelihood of sticking with these habits long-term.

Mix It Up: Add variety to your routine by trying different exercises, recipes, or relaxation techniques. Variety keeps your routine fresh and exciting.

Reward Yourself: Reward yourself for reaching milestones. Choose non-food rewards that you enjoy, such as a new book, a massage, or a day trip.

Make It Social: Combine social time with healthy activities. Invite friends for a hike, join a group fitness class, or cook healthy meals together.

7. Mindfulness and Mental Strategies

Practice Mindfulness: Engage in mindfulness practices such as meditation, yoga, or deep breathing exercises.

Mindfulness helps you stay present and reduces stress.

Set Daily Intentions: Begin each day by setting positive intentions. Focus on what you want to achieve and how you want to feel.

Affirmations: Use positive affirmations to reinforce your goals and boost self-confidence. Affirmations can shift your mindset and enhance motivation.

Reflect and Adjust: Regularly reflect on your journey, assess what's working, and make necessary adjustments. Reflection keeps you aligned with your goals.

8. Prioritize Self-Care

Allocate Time for Self-Care: Dedicate time to activities that nurture your body and mind. Self-care reduces stress and improves overall well-being.

Balance Work and Rest: Ensure a healthy balance between work, exercise, and rest. Overworking or overtraining can lead to burnout and decreased motivation.

Listen to Your Body: Pay attention to your body's signals. Rest when needed, and adjust your activities based on how you feel.

Nurture Emotional Health: Engage in activities that support your emotional health, such as spending time in nature, journaling, or seeking therapy.

9. Build a Routine with Flexibility

Create a Routine: Establish a daily routine that incorporates healthy habits. A structured routine provides stability and reduces decision fatigue.

Allow Flexibility: While routines are important, it's equally important to remain flexible. Adapt your routine as needed to accommodate changes and avoid rigidity.

Plan Ahead: Plan your meals, workouts, and self-care activities. Planning helps you stay organized and reduces the likelihood of unhealthy choices.

Stay Consistent: Consistency is key to forming lasting habits. Stick to your routine as much as possible, but be gentle with yourself when life gets in the way.

10. Seek Professional Guidance

Consult Experts: Work with healthcare professionals, nutritionists, or personal trainers who can provide personalized advice and support.

Regular Check-ins: Schedule regular check-ins with your healthcare providers to monitor your progress and make necessary adjustments.

Educational Resources: Use educational resources provided by professionals to enhance your understanding and stay motivated.

Join Programs: Enroll in health and wellness programs that offer structured guidance and community support.

Final Thoughts and Encouragement

Embarking on a journey towards a healthier lifestyle is one of the most rewarding commitments you can make for yourself. It requires dedication, patience, and a willingness to embrace change. As you continue on this path, it's essential to remain encouraged and motivated, even when challenges arise. Here are some final thoughts and words of encouragement to support you in maintaining a healthier lifestyle.

Embrace the Journey, Not Just the Destination

Focus on the Process: Understand that a healthier lifestyle is not a destination but a continuous journey. Every small step you take contributes to your overall well-being.

Celebrate Small Wins: Recognize and celebrate the small victories along the way. Whether it's choosing a healthy meal, completing a workout, or simply feeling better, each success matters.

Be Patient: Progress might be slow at times, and that's perfectly okay. Patience is key to long-term success. Trust the process and know that consistent efforts will pay off.

Enjoy the Experience: Find joy in the changes you are making. Whether it's discovering new recipes, enjoying physical activities, or connecting with like-minded individuals, savor each moment.

Cultivate a Positive Mindset

Positive Thinking: Cultivate a positive mindset by focusing on what you have achieved rather than what you have yet to accomplish. Positive thinking can significantly influence your motivation and overall outlook.

Overcome Negative Self-Talk: Challenge and reframe negative thoughts. Instead of saying, "I can't do this," try, "I am capable of making positive changes."

Practice Gratitude: Regularly reflect on the things you are grateful for. Gratitude can shift your focus from what is lacking to what is abundant in your life.

Visualize Success: Regularly visualize your success. Imagine how you will feel and the benefits you will enjoy as you achieve your health goals.

Stay Connected and Supported

Seek Support: Don't hesitate to seek support from friends, family, or professionals. Having a strong support network can provide encouragement and accountability.

Join Communities: Engage with communities or groups that share similar health goals. The shared experiences and advice can be incredibly motivating.

Share Your Journey: Share your progress and challenges with others. Whether through social media, a blog, or in person, sharing your journey can inspire and motivate both you and others.

Learn from Others: Listen to the experiences and advice of others who have successfully adopted a healthier lifestyle. Their stories can provide valuable insights and inspiration.

Adapt and Evolve

Flexibility is Key: Be flexible and open to change. Life is unpredictable, and being adaptable will help you navigate through different phases and challenges.

Learn from Setbacks: View setbacks as learning opportunities rather than failures. Analyze what went wrong, adjust your approach, and keep moving forward.

Stay Informed: Continuously educate yourself about health and wellness. Staying informed keeps you motivated and equipped with the latest knowledge to make better decisions.

Experiment and Innovate: Don't be afraid to try new things. Experiment with different types of exercises, recipes, and relaxation techniques to find what works best for you.

Prioritize Self-Care

Listen to Your Body: Pay attention to your body's needs. Rest when you need to, nourish your body with healthy foods, and take time for relaxation and recovery.

Balance and Moderation: Strive for balance and moderation in all aspects of your life. It's not about perfection, but about making sustainable and enjoyable changes.

Practice Mindfulness: Engage in mindfulness practices such as meditation, deep breathing, or yoga. Mindfulness can help reduce stress and keep you grounded.

Reward Yourself: Reward yourself for your hard work and dedication. Choose rewards that support your healthy lifestyle, such as a relaxing spa day, a new book, or a fun outing.

Look Forward with Optimism

Future Vision: Keep a clear vision of your future and how a healthier lifestyle will enhance it. This vision can serve as a powerful motivator during challenging times.

Stay Motivated: Keep finding new sources of motivation. Whether through reading inspirational stories, watching motivational videos, or setting new goals, continuously fuel your drive.

Consistency is Key: Remember that consistency is more important than intensity. Regular, small efforts can lead to significant, long-term changes.

Believe in Yourself: Have confidence in your ability to change. Believe that you are capable of achieving your health goals and living a healthier, happier life.